Zoé
You are an am...
heal...
Keep...

Chinese Medicine

& HEALTHY WEIGHT MANAGEMENT

An Evidence-based Integrated Approach

Salute'
Juliette Aiyana

By Juliette Aiyana, L.Ac.

Published by:
BLUE POPPY PRESS
A Division of Blue Poppy Enterprises, Inc.
5441 Western Ave., #2
BOULDER, CO 80301

First Edition, May 2007
Second Printing, April 2008

ISBN 1-891845-44-6
ISBN 978-1-891845-44-4
LC#2007926499

COMP Designation: Compilation of functional translations using a standard translational terminology plus an original work.

Cover and text design by Eric J. Brearton

10 9 8 7 6 5 4 3 2

Printed at Edwards Brothers, Ann Arbor, MI on recycled paper and soy inks.

Table of Contents

Acknowledgements

This book dedicated in memory of Miri Rosen-Pyros. She was a major catalyst for my career in Chinese medicine and nutritional healing.

Renee Rallo, I am profoundly grateful for you. Thank you for your assistance as my editor, writing mentor, research assistant, and especially for cowriting the glycemic index information in the book. You are my best friend, I love you, I look up to you, I am inspired by you, I learn from you, and I am challenged toward greatness by you. May you be showered with blessings.

Mom and Dad, I have inexpressible appreciation for you, for raising me in a healthy kitchen, for giving me vitamins and herbs, for taking me to the chiropractor and teaching me to critically analyze media advertisements which attempt to sway my eating habits and perception of body image, for helping set up my practice in Chinese medicine many years ago, and for your proofreading of this book and all your loving support.

Thank you to my publishers, Bob Flaws and Honora Lee Wolfe, and the entire Blue Poppy team for your encouragement, your trust in my ability, and your professionalism.

Thanks to my best friends, angels, and co-counselors, Jahna, Deyanira and Steven. We have been through thick and thin together through the decades. I possess the deepest love and respect for all of you and I am blessed to have you in my life. Corey, *tu eres mi corazon*. Thanks to Danny for encouraging me to write a book about diet. Thanks to all of my family, my Italian-American heritage, our appreciation and acceptance of various body types, and our delicious food. Our enthusiasm and enjoyment for food and gatherings with friends and family have influenced the spirit of this book and the spirit of my life.

Thanks to my office mangers who have worked with me over the years, Daisy Thompson, Laura Broomhall, and Jessica Denis. I do not know where I would be without your help compiling research for this book, taking care of all the daily details in running the office, and your loving support and enthusiasm. Thanks to Yelena Sukhodrev for your research assistance.

Thanks to all of the women with whom I worked for within the natural health community: Danielle Scallia, the first person to hire me as a massage therapist and who trusted me to manage her first spa, Kay Williams, LMT, Ilyne Kobrin, DC, and Abbi Bliss, LMT. I am lucky to have watched you run your own practices with strength, independence, love, perseverance, and dedication, and I have modeled the way I run my practice after you.

I am deeply grateful to Joshua Paynter, L.Ac., my acupuncturist, herbalist, and colleague. Our many conversations about this book, your enthusiastic support, and your academically rigorous review of drafts were all extremely valuable to me. I hold you in the highest regard. Special thanks to my colleague Jessica Silver, L.Ac. for reviewing drafts of this book and all your wonderful healing work with our patients. Special thanks also go to Patrick Sullivan, A.P. for everything. Thanks to all of my teachers at the Florida Institute of Traditional Chinese Medicine and to my professional associates: Brian Benjamin Carter, L.Ac., Mark Brinson, A.P., Tom Cristello, DC, Liz Barbera, L.Ac., and Janet Tsai, L.Ac. Many thanks to Anne-Marie Colbin; had it not been for the powerful influence of your books, I may never have written this one. *Metta* to all my Dharma teachers, including His Holiness the Dalai Llama, Eric Butterworth, Geshe Jigme Gyatso, Sharon Salzberg, Pema Chodron, Geshe Michael Roach, and Sandra Weinberg and to the Dharma organizations Tibet House and New York Insight Meditation.

Thanks especially to all of my patients and students who have taught me to be a better practitioner, communicator, and writer, who inspired much of the content of this book, who waited patiently for and encouraged me to complete this book, and who have taught me 1001 invaluable lessons. I wake up every day with a smile on my face, feeling like I am the luckiest woman in the world because I work for you.

Foreword

Eating is the most fundamental means that we have toward a cultivating a healthy body. There should be no need for sophisticated methodologies for discerning what is good to eat and when we've had too much or too little. We either feel good or we don't, or we feel hungry or satiated. It would seem that these should be self evident truths, but for some reason this is not so. We eat for reasons beyond sustenance, we eat foods that, were it not for laboratories and industry, would not otherwise exist. As such, people around the globe are faced with the crises of obesity, heart disease, diabetes, etc., all in rates unrivaled in history. In answer to this, modern scientific methods have been employed by various researchers, professional nutritionists, and doctors in order to develop a variety of means for people to employ in controlling their weight, having more energy, and minimizing the risks associated with poor eating habits, poor foods or both. The result of this endeavor most often comes in the form of a specific diet, which in the end is much like an eating protocol. These diets are usually born out of studies of particular aspects of food, like fats and carbohydrates, and their behavior within the dynamics of metabolism and the resulting effects on health and well being. The diet is then formed around this outcome oriented kernel. The effect of the specific diet is then generalized to represent all humans who share the same physiology.

People, looking for the next solution to their dissatisfaction with body size or health, turn to this latest scientific phenomenon in hopes of finally achieving their dietary goals. For some there is incredible success, but for others there is abject failure and frustration. Why would there be differences in the effects of this diet when the research and data would suggest that success is a guarantee?

How can a diet be right for some and not for others? This is not likely do to any shortcoming in the studies that form the basis for the diet, or any shortcoming in the diets themselves. Rather this reflects that there must be some other factor in the proper implementation of the diet, or particular food type. Beside the obvious differences in dieters will power, there must be something in the reality of each individual human themselves that governs the outcomes of particular eating habits. From the obvious "she eats whatever she wants and never gains a pound" to the more subtle realities of health and well being, we are all aware of how differently we respond to foods.

This recognition of the differences in constitution, or physiological patterning, called pattern diagnosis, is one of the defining characteristics of Chinese medicine. The key to integrating Chinese medicine into the Western dialogue concerning diet lies within the methodology of pattern diagnosis. Recognizing that all people are not going to respond similarly to a given diet or food type, is an invaluable asset to discerning what choices would best suit a patients needs. The nutrition books and guidelines need not be rewritten or reorganized; the food pyramid need not be inverted. We simply need to observe the nuance of each individual's constitution and react to these signs appropriately. Standing firmly upon the foundation of sound scientific research, with the accumulated experience of Chinese medical diagnostics and the related implementation of food types, we are in good position to deliver excellent care to our patients. We can help them to find a diet that will be consistent with their particular needs, and give them both the care and tools to be successful in achieving their goals. Toward this end, Juliette Aiyana has put together a most valuable tool by writing this book. A tool that accounts for both modern scientific understandings of nutrition and diet, particular attributes of pattern diagnosis and the energetics of foods according to Chinese food and drug taxonomies. This book is of great value to both the practitioner and the patient, and furthermore should be found very soon within the curriculum of Chinese medicine schools. As the spirit of "integration" takes the place of "alternative" and "complimentary" we will be in increasingly greater need of books that value the traditions and methods of Chinese medicine, while reflecting the great strides made by scientific research. I believe this book does this well, and, as a result, our field is all the better because of this spirit of respect for science and pride in our own traditional methods.

Joshua M. Paynter, L.Ac., Professor of Chinese Medicine, Touro College
New York, April 2007

Preface

In my clinical practice, I treat weight loss patients on a daily basis. Many patients present with weight loss as their chief or secondary complaint. Some of them come in with preconceptions about how acupuncture is used to treat weight loss. They often ask, "Is it true that ear tacks can make you lose weight?" This question reveals their hopeful assumption that acupuncture provides a quick fix to their weight loss problems. With a friendly smile, I gently respond, "No, unfortunately there is no magic bullet for weight loss; no one magic ear or body acupoint will melt away the pounds. If it did, I would be a fabulously rich woman with a line of patients stretching from New York to California! However, the good news is that a holistic approach to weight loss, including acupuncture, Chinese herbs, diet, and exercise is very successful. Many of my weight loss patients lose an average of 10 percent of body weight (5-15 pounds) in 2-3 months. But first, you have to become committed to making changes in lifestyle, and, during our treatment sessions, I'll counsel you on making and maintaining these changes."

This manual is about the integrated Chinese-Western medical treatment of overweight and obesity. I have written it so that practitioners of acupuncture and Chinese medicine can immediately integrate the best of Chinese medicine with the most up-to-date insights of biomedical weight loss research. Within this book, readers will find acupuncture, Chinese herbal, and Chinese dietary protocols, modern nutritional therapies, and modern exercise research and therapy along with the National Institutes for Health (NIH) guidelines for the assessment and treatment of overweight and obesity as well as guidelines from the Centers for Disease Control (CDC) and the American Heart Association (AHA). Rather than trying to reinvent the wheel by rewriting or reformatting existing guidelines for the treatment of overweight and obesity, I sought out and was granted permission by the NIH and AHA to include large amounts of information they have already published for the purposes of educating both practitioners and patients. Most of the healthy eating and exercise tips contained in this text are geared for practitioners treating adult (not pediatric) weight loss and the prevention of weight gain. Though primarily written for practitioners, this book may also be read and used by patients being treated for overweight and obesity or those who simply seek a healthy lifestyle in general.

I have been in clinical practice in the natural health field since 1992. Before becoming a Chinese medical practitioner, I was a massage therapist for nearly a decade. Over the years, I have engaged in thousands of conversations with patients about wellness, health maintenance, diet, exercise, the mind-body connection, behavioral change, and more. Through these conversations, I have learned that such patient-practitioner dialogue supports and strengthens the effectiveness of treatment. Such conversations empower patients through education about their treatment and how they can engage as proactive participants in their healing and wellness. Happily, over the years, I have learned how to communicate the Chinese medical paradigm to Western patients. In fact, I do this so well that many of my patients begin to speak to me using Chinese medical terminology. They even know what Chinese medical patterns their herb formulas are treating. So when Blue Poppy asked me to write a practice manual on weight loss for acupuncturists and Chinese medical practitioners, I knew that I would write a book not just about which points and herbs to use for each pattern but also about how to treat the patient as a whole, how to communicate with them in a language they understand while teaching them to speak about themselves and their treatment in the language of Chinese medicine. It is my wish that this practice manual may be helpful to those in clinical practice who are trying to create a truly authentic and practical integrative healing partnership with their patients. May the information contained in this book inspire your practice no matter what the patient's main complaint and may this book serve as a tool for patient education and empowerment.

Juliette Aiyana, L.Ac.

Introduction

The scope of the problem

According the NIH (National Institutes of Health), 97 million American adults are overweight or obese.[1] Breaking this down, 58 million are overweight, 40 million are obese, and three million are morbidly obese.[2] Eight out of 10 Americans over 25 are overweight. Seventy-eight percent of Americans are not meeting basic activity level recommendations, while 25 percent are completely sedentary. In addition, there is a 76 percent increase in type 2 diabetes in adults 30-40 years old since 1990.

> **Eight out of 10 Americans over 25 are overweight.**

The NIH and the CDC (Centers for Disease Control) state that obesity is the second leading cause of preventable death in the United States. (Cigarette smoking related death is the leading cause.) This increase in weight gain is found throughout the world in industrialized countries where there is a rise in consumption of processed and so-called fastfoods combined with sedentary jobs and lifestyles. For instance, in China, approximately 90 million adults are clinically defined as overweight or obese and that number is expected to double in the next decade. In the United States as in most developing countries, cardiovascular disease is the number one killer of women, and obesity contributes to cardiovascular disease as a comorbidity factor. According to the

[1] NIH Executive Summary: *Clinical Guidelines On The Identification, Evaluation, And Treatment of Overweight And Obesity In Adults*, p vii

[2] Obesity Statistics, http://www.annecollins.com/obesity/statistics-obesity.htm accessed 1.25.07

AHA (American Heart Association), "Lifestyle approaches to prevent cardio-vascular disease (CVD), such as smoking cessation, regular exercise, weight management, and a heart-healthy diet, are Class I recommendations for all women and therefore should be a top priority in clinical practice." [3]

Not only are overweight and obesity becoming more and more common in developed countries, this pandemic is also placing a growing burden on these societies. For instance, as the prevalence of overweight and obesity has increased in the United States, so have related health care costs—both direct and indirect. Direct health care costs refer to preventive, diagnostic, and treatment services such as physician visits, medications, and hospital and nursing home care. Indirect costs are the value of wages lost by people unable to work because of illness or disability, as well as the value of future earnings lost by premature death. A recent study estimated annual medical spending due to overweight and obesity (BMI ≥ 25) to be as much as $92.6 billion dollars in 2002 —9.1 percent of U.S. health expenditures. In addition, there are the costs of lost productivity due to obesity. In 1994, these were estimated to be $3.9 billion for Americans 17-64 years of age.[4]

The role of Chinese medicine in helping solve this problem

Practitioners of Chinese medicine in North America, Europe, and other non-Asian countries are often our patients' main source for health care and health information. We are usually the health care provider who spends the most amount of time with the patient. The average medical doctor in the UK spends only 10 minutes consulting with the patient, and this amount of time is likely the same if not less in the U.S.[5] In my experience, practitioners of Chinese medicine usually spend an average of 1.5 hours with each patient on the first visit. Of this, one hour or more is the consultation and the remaining 30 minutes are for the acupuncture treatment, while follow-up visits average 40 minutes (10 minutes talk and 30 minutes acupuncture). This means that our patients have time to ask us plenty of questions about self-care and the treatments we administer. During this time, practitioners can educate and counsel our patients on diet, exercise, self-care therapies, and other lifestyle changes. In fact, it is my experience that effective weight loss treatment depends on all types of health care providers, including Chinese medical practitioners, medical doctors, nutritionists, and fitness profession-

---

[3] Mosca *et al.*, "Evidence-Based Guidelines for Cardiovascular Disease in Women," *Circulation*.2004;109: 672-693

[4] http://win.niddk.nih.gov/statistics/index.htm#other accessed 1.25.07

[5] Deveugele, M. *et al.*, "Consultation Length In General Practice: Cross Sectional Study In Six European Countries," *BMJ*. 2002;325:472 (31 August)

als, to maintain consistent contact with and to monitor the patient. In addition to acupuncture, diet, exercise, and behavioral change are integral for success for weight loss and maintenance. Therefore, in this book, Chinese medical treatment, diet, and exercise are each discussed in separate chapters, while suggestions for behavioral change are integrated throughout. Therefore, this book discusses all aspects of treatment. Also included are many references for patients and practitioners to find out even more information on all aspects of weight loss treatment, including when and to whom to refer patients for integrative care.

Finding out the real problem

When a patient comes in saying that she or he wants to lose weight, the first thing I do is to find out why. During our initial conversation, I try to explore the patient's motivation for weight loss to understand if that desire is truly reasonable. Some patients are within or sadly below his or her healthy body mass index (BMI), yet they still desire to be thinner. In other cases, I may find out that the patient is actually anorexic or bulimic. When patients who are at a healthy weight or are underweight seek weight-loss treatment, I try to understand the root of his or her desire. We talk about her[6] perception of weight, her body, and her culture. I often find that these patients worry because their body has changed shape over the course of their lives. However, the truth is that the human body is naturally prone to change with age regardless of sex. Therefore, I often remind my female patients that, "We are women. Our bodies change shape and tend to become more curvaceous as we age. In most cultures, these curves are considered beautiful, healthy, and a sign of fertility or wisdom." If the patient is at a healthy BMI, she should just keep up the good work. I often tell my healthy patients: "You are healthy. I don't see anything wrong. Keep doing what you're doing. I will support your goal in weight loss as long as you stay within your BMI, but rest assured that you are a healthy woman." Sometimes, when a mirror is held by a compassionate other, we may suddenly see reality or at least open to its possibility. Once my patients see themselves in such a compassionate mirror, I then give them some practical health tips and suggestions for how to prepare for future changes in body type and health. On the other hand, many overweight or obese patients sensibly seek treatment for weight loss and obesity-related health risks or disease, such as diabetes. Thus I also counsel them for weight loss to help reduce the comorbidity factor.

---

[6] Unfortunately, it is a fact of clinical practice that most patients who are anorexic or bulimic are female.

No simple solutions

As the *NIH Executive Summary* states;

Obesity is a complex multifactorial chronic disease that develops from an interaction of genotype and the environment. Our understanding of how and why obesity develops is incomplete but involves the integration of social, behavioral, cultural, physiological, metabolic and genetic factors.

In the Tang dynasty, Sun Si-miao, the greatest Chinese doctor of his time said that the Chinese medical practitioner should first modify the patient's diet and lifestyle and, only if those remedies are not enough, should they go on to administer acupuncture and Chinese herbal medicine. As an extension of this, I find that Chinese medical treatments are most effective when integrated with modern medical treatments and advice.

While there is agreement about the health risks of overweight and obesity, there is less agreement about their management. Some have argued against treating obesity because of the difficulty in maintaining long-term weight loss and of potentially negative consequences of the frequently seen pattern of weight cycling in obese subjects.[7]

Because Chinese medicine is a comprehensive health care system, it has a history of successfully treating a variety of both acute and chronic disease through a combination of professionally administered therapies and balancing lifestyle and environmental factors with the patient's constitutional (*i.e.*, genetic) factors with which they were born. Thus, in many ways, Chinese medicine is already akin to the NIH guidelines set forth for the treatment of overweight and obesity. For instance, in the Tang dynasty, Sun Si-miao, the greatest Chinese doctor of his time said that the Chinese medical practitioner should first modify the patient's diet and lifestyle and, only if those remedies are not enough, should they go on to administer acupuncture and Chinese herbal medicine. As an extension of this, I find that Chinese medical treatments are most effective when integrated with modern medical treatments and advice. Chinese medicine offers a variety of safe and effective treatments which can be easily integrated with evidence-based diet and exercise therapies. Evidence shows that the most effective treatment for overweight and obesity are a combination of dietary change (to lower calorie and lower fat diets), changes in exercise behavior patterns, and overall behavior

---

[7] NIH Executive Summary, *op cit.* p vii

change therapy, or, as we practitioners of Chinese medicine would say, lifestyle changes. In my experience, when we add such effective professionally administered therapies as acupuncture and Chinese herbal medicine to these other proven therapies, our patients get an even better result.

What's reasonable to expect

Weight-loss treatment goals should aim to reduce a reasonable and moderate amount of body weight. In fact, most NIH trials and Chinese medical research alike find an average of about 8-10% of baseline weight loss to be common among weight-loss patients. Additionally, weight management treatment goals include the long-term maintenance of healthy/healthier body weight and the prevention of future weight gain. In my experience, losing weight over a sustained period of time is safer than crash diets, over-the-counter (OTC) weight loss aids or supplements, prescription medications, and surgery, and weight loss can be sustained for a longer time if the patient continues weight-loss management goals using self-care techniques, such as diet, exercise, and stress reduction.

Being overweight as a cofactor in other diseases

While being overweight may be the patient's primary complaint, being overweight is a risk factor for the development of a number of other diseases. In the last decade or so, Western medical practitioners have identified a condition called metabolic syndrome (a.k.a. Kaplan's syndrome and syndrome X). This is a combination of being overweight (especially being overweight in one's trunk), insulin resistance, hypertension, and high cholesterol. This condition is known to be a risk factor for the eventual development of cardiovascular disease and increases one's chances of dying from heart attack and stroke. Being overweight is also a cofactor for the development of diabetes mellitus along with all its comorbidities, such as various neuropathies, vascular disease, macular degeneration, and kidney disease. In fact, many of our weight-loss patients present with a variety of these other diseases.

80% of type 2 diabetes is related to obesity

70% of cardiovascular disease is related to obesity

42% breast and colon cancer is diagnosed among obese individuals

30% of gallbladder surgery is related to obesity

26% of obese people have high blood pressure[8]

---

[8] http://www.annecollins.com/obesity/statistics-obesity.htm accessed 1.25.07

Therefore, it is important for us to treat both the root cause of their condition as well as its branch symptoms or associated diseases. To do this knowledgebly and responsibly, we need to take into consideration the patient's BMI, waist circumference, waist-to-hip ratio, and any other concomitant diseases or other risk factors in crafting our overall treatment plan. Therefore, practitioners may need to refer to other specialty manuals on cardiovascular disease, diabetes, and nephrology. To be ignorant of these things risks failure or even making the patient's situation worse. In other words, when patients come to us saying that they want to lose weight, we need to look at their entire medical situation and not just focus on weight loss.

Quick fixes to be avoided

In extreme cases, many patients choose or are counseled by their Western medical doctors to use surgery or pharmacotherapy to treat weight issues. If your patients are considering surgery, I strongly suggest they get a second opinion from another MD. They also should be well-informed by the MD of all the possible short and long-term side effects. For instance, it seems that liposuction has less short- and long-term risk factors then does gastrointestinal surgery if the patient suffers from simple obesity. However, the risk factors of liposuction rise when the patient is either extremely obese, at a healthy BMI, or underweight.

The use of some weight-loss drugs has proven fatal over the years. Many women have died of heart failure from lethal combinations of drugs which have been subsequently outlawed. Nevertheless, even today, there are many drugs which still carry great risks of heart disease and addiction. Though health-related problems prompt some patients to take weight-loss drugs, societal pressure, low self-worth, and poor self-image are common reasons that many patients take potentially dangerous drugs for weight loss. When a patient like this seeks treatment from us for weight loss, we have the chance to help them change their view of self. In such cases, we can help them reduce stress and depression with acupuncture and Chinese herbal medicine and refer them for counseling.

If a patient does decide to use prescription weight-loss drugs or surgery, the patient still risks gaining weight back afterwards if they do not change their diet and lifestyle. Therefore, even with drug and/or surgical treatment, there should be an integrated diet, exercise, social and behavioral therapeutic support system, and overall health maintenance program in place over the duration of treatment and in the long term after the surgical or drug treatment. In my experience, acupuncture and Chinese medicine can fit in very well in such an overall integrated treatment plan.

Speaking compassionately with patients

During inquiry and counseling, practition- | The words we use among ers should remember that our word is our | ourselves and with those wand, and I believe we should always take | whom we counsel is very care to use terminology which empowers | important to the relationship our patients. If a patient has been diag- | we develop with patients. nosed with arthritis, we tell the patient, "You have arthritis." We do not say, "You are arthritis." When we say, "You *have* arthritis," it separates the patient from the disease. When we say things like, "You are fat," the patient thinks they *are* the disease. Practitioners of Chinese medicine know that people are not their diseases but rather that the root cause of the disease is based on a variety of causes and conditions. I will use the word "fat" interchangeably with the clinical term "adipose tissue." However, I never use the term "fat person." "Fat person" is a derogative term in most English-speaking cultures. I have read English translations of Chinese obesity studies using the term "fat person." For example, they may say, "Fat people have dampness." Instead, I use the clinically defined terms "overweight" (BMI 25 – 29.9), "obese" (Class 1, BMI 30-34.9, Class 2, BMI 35-39.9), or "extreme obesity" (Class 3, BMI greater than or equal to 40).

Many patients prefer to hear the term "excess weight" than "obese" during counseling. The term "excess weight" reduces the chance of the patient taking the description personally by separating them from the manifestation of the disease. Encouragement, not embarrassment, is the best clinical choice in this matter. I encourage all of my patients to love and respect their bodies no matter what. In fact, one of my patients remarked on the difference in hearing me use the term excess weight instead of obesity because being categorized as obese by her MD made her feel doomed to remain in that category. Being described as a person who has excess weight, on the other hand, made her feel capable of changing that condition. The words we use among ourselves and with those whom we counsel is very important to the relationship we develop with patients. Therefore, I make a point to empower the patient's role in self-care by fostering a nonjudgmental discourse with the patient and with my colleagues.

Putting it all together

Many of our obese patients are facing serious health consequences. When faced with a health crisis, patients face the reality that many aspects of life must change. This can be a daunting or overwhelming challenge. Some may face their unwillingness to change, fear of change, or attachment to the out-come. Others may be unable to let go of old habits or may lack the will to do so. Many feel hopeless. Some hope for a magic weight-loss bullet, that secret ear tack, acupoint, or herb which will cause them to lose pounds effortlessly without self-care. However, our patients should be counseled that Chinese medicine requires self-care and lifestyle change in combination with acupuncture and herbs in order to be truly successful. To lose weight and keep it off, patients must transform their diet, their lifestyle, and their way of thinking and schedule time for home cooking, exercise, acupuncture visits, and taking their herbs regularly. In addition, I always encourage them to have fun and enjoy life.

The approach presented in this book is simply to apply standard Chinese medical diagnostics and treatments integrated with exercise, modern nutritional sense, and NIH recommendations. If you choose to incorporate the information contained in this book into your practice, I hope and trust you will adapt the acupuncture points, herbs, and nutritional and exercise suggestions for your patient's unique Chinese medical patterns and overall medical situation. One of the real strong points of Chinese medicine is its ability to customize treatment for each individual patient. The protocols given in this book are only models or starting places, but you have a unique human patient in front of you. As master martial artist Bruce Lee said, "Research your own experience. Absorb what is useful. Reject what is useless. Add what is specifically your own."

Obesity Assessment & Management 2

The ancient books on Chinese medicine do not provide practitioners with much specific guidance for the assessment and management of obesity because obesity was not the health epidemic that it has become to modern medicine. Hence, the vast majority of information in this chapter is excerpted from the National Institutes of Health's Practical Guide: *Identification, Evaluation and Treatment of Overweight and Obesity in Adults*. The NIH created this guide for the purpose of free reprint and distribution amongst health care providers. The entire guide is freely downloadable from the NIH website in order to fulfill the NIH's mission to advance practitioner education and participation in the treatment of overweight and obesity. I recommend that all practitioners read the manual in its entirety. I have provided bracketed commentary in some segments of the guidelines, often indicating the practitioner should refer to the NIH guide for more information. The few paragraphs in this chapter that I personally have added begin with my initials in brackets [JA].

The NIH makes clear that, "Treatment of overweight or obesity incorporates a two step process: assessment and management."

Assessment includes determination of the degree of obesity and overall health status. Management involves not only weight loss and maintenance of body weight but also measures to control other risk factors. Obesity is a chronic disease; patient and practitioner must understand that successful treatment requires a lifelong effort. Convincing evidence supports the benefit of weight loss for reducing blood pressure, lowering blood glucose, and improving dyslipi-demias.[9]

In the year 2000, the NIH estimated that 97 million adults in the United States are overweight or obese, a condition that substantially raises their risk of morbidity from hypertension, dyslipidemia, type 2 diabetes, coronary heart disease, stroke, gallbladder disease, osteoarthritis, sleep apnea and respiratory problems, and endometrial, breast, prostate, and colon cancers. Higher body weights are also associated with increases in all-cause mortality. Obese individuals may also suffer from social stigmatization and discrimination. In overweight patients, control of cardiovascular risk factors deserves equal emphasis as weight reduction therapy. As the second leading cause of preventable death in the United States today, overweight and obesity pose a major public health challenge.[10]

According to the U.S. Surgeon General, "Solely having a BMI in the overweight or obese range does not necessarily indicate that a person is unhealthy. Other risk factors, such as high blood pressure, high cholesterol, smoking, diabetes, and personal and family medical history are important to consider when assessing overall health."[11]

NIH Assessment Guidelines

Body mass index

Assessment of a patient should include the evaluation of body mass index (BMI), waist circumference, and overall medical risk. To estimate BMI, multiply the individual's weight (in pounds) by 703, and then divide by the height (in inches) squared. This approximates BMI in kilograms per meter squared (kg/m^2). There is evidence to support the use of BMI in risk assessment since it provides a more accurate measure of total body fat compared with the assessment of body weight alone. Neither bioelectric impedance nor height-weight tables provide an advantage over BMI in the clinical management of all adult patients, regardless of gender. Clinical judgment must be employed when evaluating very muscular patients because BMI may overestimate the degree of fatness in these patients.

[Muscle mass weighs more than fat weighs. Patients who regularly

---

[9] NIH Practical Guide: *Identification, Evaluation and Treatment of Overweight and Obesity in Adults*, p. 1
[10] NIH Executive Summary: *Clinical Guidelines on the Identification, Evaluation and Treatment of Overweight and Obesity in Adults*, p. vii
[11] http://www.surgeongeneral.gov/topics/obesity/calltoaction/fact_advice.htm accessed 10.19.06

engage in weight-training exercise will gain muscle weight and may mistakenly think they have gained fat, encountering a set back. In this case, advise them that the training likely resulted in a muscle mass weight gain which is positive achievement representing health and strength. They should assess weight gains and losses by observing their changing body shape and how clothing fits, not just by weighing themselves on a scale.]

The recommended classifications for BMI have been adopted by the Expert Panel on the Identification, Evaluation, and Treatment of Overweight and Obesity in Adults and have been endorsed by leading organizations of health professionals.
(*See the following two pages.*)

Waist circumference

Excess abdominal fat is an important, independent risk factor for disease. The evaluation of waist circumference to assess the risks associated with obesity or overweight is supported by research. The measurement of waist-to-hip ratio provides no advantage over waist circumference alone. Waist circumference measurement is particularly useful in patients who are categorized as normal or overweight. It is not necessary to measure waist circumference in individuals with BMI's $\geq$ 35 kg/m2 since it adds little to the predictive power of the disease risk classification of BMI. Men who have waist circumferences greater than 40 inches, and women who have waist circumferences greater than 35 inches, are at higher risk of diabetes, dyslipidemia, hypertension, and cardiovascular disease because of excess abdominal fat. Individuals with waist circumferences greater than these values should be considered one risk category above that defined by their BMI. The relationship between BMI and waist circumference for defining risk is shown in Table 2 on page 10 [refer to NIH guide].

> Men who have waist circumferences greater than 40 inches, and women who have waist circumferences greater than 35 inches, are at higher risk of diabetes, dyslipidemia, hypertension, and cardiovascular disease because of excess abdominal fat.

Practitioners who wish to employ this diagnostic tool in clinical practice must first refer to the NIH guide which includes illustrative directions on how to take the measurements.

[JA] During assessment, practitioners should adhere to the above standards and refrain from diagnosing patients based upon outdated methods, personal preference of body type, or snap, nonevidence based judgment. Our patients have feelings which deserve to be taken into account, and their perception of our and society's judgments contribute to patients' motivation for self-

Appendix A. Body Mass Index Table

Body Weight (pounds)

BMI	19	20	21	22	23	24	25	26	27	28	29	30	31	32	33	34	35
Height (inches)																	
58	91	96	100	105	110	115	119	124	129	134	138	143	148	153	158	162	167
59	94	99	104	109	114	119	124	128	133	138	143	148	153	158	163	168	173
60	97	102	107	112	118	123	128	133	138	143	148	153	158	163	168	174	179
61	100	106	111	116	122	127	132	137	143	148	153	158	164	169	174	180	185
62	104	109	115	120	126	131	136	142	147	153	158	164	169	175	180	186	191
63	107	113	118	124	130	135	141	146	152	158	163	169	175	180	186	191	197
64	110	116	122	128	134	140	145	151	157	163	169	174	180	186	192	197	204
65	114	120	126	132	138	144	150	156	162	168	174	180	186	192	198	204	210
66	118	124	130	136	142	148	155	161	167	173	179	186	192	198	204	210	216
67	121	127	134	140	146	153	159	166	172	178	185	191	198	204	211	217	223
68	125	131	138	144	151	158	164	171	177	184	190	197	203	210	216	223	230
69	128	135	142	149	155	162	169	176	182	189	196	203	209	216	223	230	236
70	132	139	146	153	160	167	174	181	188	195	202	209	216	222	229	236	243
71	136	143	150	157	165	172	179	186	193	200	208	215	222	229	236	243	250
72	140	147	154	162	169	177	184	191	199	206	213	221	228	235	242	250	258
73	144	151	159	166	174	182	189	197	204	212	219	227	235	242	250	257	265
74	148	155	163	171	179	186	194	202	210	218	225	233	241	249	256	264	272
75	152	160	168	176	184	192	200	208	216	224	232	240	248	256	264	272	279
76	156	164	172	180	189	197	205	213	221	230	238	246	254	263	271	279	287

BMI	36	37	38	39	40	41	42	43	44	45	46	47	48	49	50	51	52	53	54
58	172	177	181	186	191	196	201	205	210	215	220	224	229	234	239	244	248	253	258
59	178	183	188	193	198	203	208	212	217	222	227	232	237	242	247	252	257	262	267
60	184	189	194	199	204	209	215	220	225	230	235	240	245	250	255	261	266	271	276
61	190	195	201	206	211	217	222	227	232	238	243	248	254	259	264	269	275	280	285
62	196	202	207	213	218	224	229	235	240	246	251	256	262	267	273	278	284	289	295
63	203	208	214	220	225	231	237	242	248	254	259	265	270	276	282	287	293	299	304
64	209	215	221	227	232	238	244	250	256	262	267	273	279	285	291	296	302	308	314
65	216	222	228	234	240	246	252	258	264	270	276	282	288	294	300	306	312	318	324
66	223	229	235	241	247	253	260	266	272	278	284	291	297	303	309	315	322	328	334
67	230	236	242	249	255	261	268	274	280	287	293	299	306	312	319	325	331	338	344
68	236	243	249	256	262	269	276	282	289	295	302	308	315	322	328	335	341	348	354
69	243	250	257	263	270	277	284	291	297	304	311	318	324	331	338	345	351	358	365
70	250	257	264	271	278	285	292	299	306	313	320	327	334	341	348	355	362	369	376
71	257	265	272	279	286	293	301	308	315	322	329	336	343	351	358	365	372	379	386
72	265	272	279	287	294	302	309	316	324	331	338	346	353	361	368	375	383	390	397
73	272	280	288	295	302	310	318	325	333	340	348	355	363	371	378	386	393	401	408
74	280	287	295	303	311	319	326	334	342	350	358	365	373	381	389	396	404	412	420
75	287	295	303	311	319	327	335	343	351	359	367	375	383	391	399	407	415	423	431
76	295	304	312	320	328	336	344	353	361	369	377	385	394	402	410	418	426	435	443

care and self-image. The following example of the effect a practitioner's words have on a patient comes directly from a clinical encounter with a patient. A female patient, aged 27, came to me very distressed and on the verge of tears after a yearly physical with her medical doctor. The MD assessed her weight by directing her to wrap her right hand around her left wrist. The tips of her fingers were unable to touch and he coldly declared her as "morbidly obese." She was hurt by his words and callous bedside manner. She told me that her self-image had been shattered. However, I uncovered the truth that, although she was overweight, she was not obese. I assured her that she need not worry that she is obese. Then I counseled her on how to eat well and exercise to maintain her health and lose the excess weight. The media and society-at-large do a good enough job indoctrinating women (and, to some degree, men) to cultivate distorted self-images. Therefore, as health care practitioners, we must responsibly diagnosis obesity based upon nothing other than the evidence-based techniques set forth by the NIH or other health education authorities.

Risk factors & comorbidities

Overall risk must take into account the potential presence of other risk factors. Some diseases or risk factors associated with obesity place patients at a high absolute risk for subsequent mortality; these will require aggressive management. Other conditions associated with obesity are less lethal but still require treatment. Those diseases or conditions that denote high absolute risk are established coronary heart disease, other atherosclerotic diseases, type 2 diabetes, and sleep apnea. Osteoarthritis, gallstones, stress incontinence, and gynecological abnormalities such as amenorrhea and menorrhagia increase risk but are not generally life-threatening. Three or more of the following risk factors also confer high absolute risk: hypertension, cigarette smoking, high low-density lipoprotein cholesterol, low high-density lipoprotein cholesterol, impaired fasting glucose, family history of early cardiovascular disease and age (male ≥ 45 years, female ≥ 55 years). The integrated approach to assessment and management is portrayed in Figure 4 on pages 16–17 of the NIH guide.[See the Bibliography.]

Readiness to lose weight

The decision to attempt weight-loss treatment should also consider the patient's readiness to make the necessary lifestyle changes. Evaluation of readiness should include the following:

- Reasons and motivation for weight loss
- Previous attempts at weight loss

- Support expected from family and friends
- Understanding of risks and benefits
- Attitudes toward physical activity
- Time availability
- Potential barriers, including financial
  limitations, to the patient's adoption of change

NIH Management Guidelines

Weight loss

Individuals at lesser risk should be counseled about effective lifestyle changes to prevent any further weight gain. Goals of therapy are to reduce body weight and maintain a lower body weight for the long term; the prevention of further weight gain is the minimum goal. An initial weight loss of 10 percent of body weight achieved over six months is a recommended target.

> After the first six months of weight-loss therapy, the priority should be weight maintenance achieved through combined changes in diet, physical activity, and behavior.

The rate of weight loss should be one to two pounds each week. Greater rates of weight loss do not achieve better long-term results. After the first six months of weight loss therapy, the priority should be weight maintenance achieved through combined changes in diet, physical activity, and behavior. Further weight loss can be considered after a period of weight maintenance.

Prevention of weight gain

In some patients, weight loss or a reduction in body fat is not achievable. A goal for these patients should be the prevention of further weight gain. Prevention of weight gain is also an appropriate goal for people with a BMI of 25 to 29.9 who are not otherwise at high risk.

Therapies

A combination of diet modification, increased physical activity, and behavior therapy can be effective.

Dietary therapy

Caloric intake should be reduced by 500 to 1,000 calories per day (kcal/day) from the current level. Most overweight and obese people should adopt long-term nutritional adjustments to reduce caloric intake.

Dietary therapy includes instructions for modifying diets to achieve this goal. Moderate caloric reduction is the goal for the majority of cases; however, diets with greater caloric deficits are used during active weight loss. The diet should be low in calories, but it should not be too low. [In other words the diet should be no less than 800 kcal/day.]

Diets

Weight loss therapy is recommended for patients with a BMI ≥ 30 and for patients with a BMI between 25-29.9 or a high-risk waist circumference, [with] two or more risk factors. Lower than 800 kcal/day have been found to be no more effective than low-calorie diets in producing weight loss. They should not be used routinely, especially not by providers untrained in their use. In general, diets containing 1,000 to 1,200 kcal/day should be selected for most women; a diet between 1,200 kcal/day and 1,600 kcal/day should be chosen for men and may be appropriate for women who weigh 165 pounds or more, or who exercise.

Long-term changes in food choices are more likely to be successful when the patient's preferences are taken into account and when the patient is educated about food composition, labeling, preparation, and portion size. Although dietary fat is a rich source of calories, reducing dietary fat without reducing calories will not produce weight loss. Frequent contact with practitioners during the period of diet adjustment is likely to improve compliance.

Physical activity

Physical activity has direct and indirect benefits. Increased physical activity is important in efforts to lose weight because it increases energy expenditure and plays an integral role in weight maintenance. Physical activity also reduces the risk of heart disease more than that achieved by weight loss alone. In addition, increased physical activity may help reduce body fat and prevent the decrease in muscle mass often found during weight loss.

For the obese patient, activity should generally be increased slowly, with care taken to avoid injury. A wide variety of activities and/or household chores, including walking, dancing, gardening, and team or individual sports, may help satisfy this goal. All adults should set a long-term goal to accumulate at least 30 minutes or more of moderate-intensity physical activity on most, and preferably all, days of the week.

Behavior therapy

Including behavioral therapy helps with compliance. Behavior therapy is a useful adjunct to planned adjustments in food intake and physical activity. Specific behavioral strategies include the following: self-monitoring, stress management, stimulus control, problem-solving, contingency management, cognitive restructuring, and social support.

Behavioral therapies may be employed to promote adoption of diet and activity adjustments; these will be useful for a combined approach to therapy. Strong evidence supports the recommendation that weight loss and weight maintenance programs should employ a combination of low-calorie diets, increased physical activity, and behavior therapy.

Pharmacotherapy

Pharmacotherapy may be helpful for eligible high-risk patients. Pharmacotherapy, approved by the FDA for long-term treatment, can be a helpful adjunct for the treatment of obesity in some patients. These drugs should be used only in the context of a treatment program that includes the elements described previously—diet, physical activity changes, and behavior therapy. If lifestyle changes do not promote weight loss after six months, drugs should be considered. Pharmacotherapy is currently limited to those patients who have a BMI ≥ 30, or those who have a BMI ≥ 27 if concomitant obesity-related risk factor or diseases exist. However, not all patients respond to a given drug. If a patient has not lost 4.4 pounds (2 kg) after four weeks, it is not likely that this patient will benefit from the drug. Currently, sibutramine and orlistat are approved by the FDA for long-term use in weight loss. Sibutramine is an appetite suppressant that is proposed to work via norepinephrine and seroton-ergic mechanisms in the brain. Orlistat inhibits fat absorption from the intestine. Both of these drugs have side effects. Sibutramine may increase blood pressure and induce tachycardia; orlistat may reduce the absorption of fat-soluble vitamins and nutrients. The decision to add a drug to an obesity treatment program should be made after consideration of all potential risks and benefits and only after all behavioral options have been exhausted.

[JA] Appetite suppressants are typically close to amphetamines (*i.e.,* "speed") in chemical structure. In the U.S., these include such drugs as Ionamin®, Fastin®, Adipex-P®, Tenuate®, and Zantryl®. Other diet pills in this category are Plegine®, Prelu-2®, Sanorex®, Didrex®, and Bontril®, and some of these may be habit forming. Outside the U.S., these include such drugs as Duromine, Linyl, Minobese, Mirapront, Normaform, Obenix, Oby-Cap, Oby-Trim, Panbesy Nyscaps, and Umine. These are the same class of drugs sold on the streets as "uppers" like cocaine. The side effects of these popular appetite suppressants include blurred vision, increased blood pressure, chest pain, heart palpitations, swelling of the legs, dizziness, dry mouth, sleeplessness, irritability, and stomach upset or constipation.

Fat-blockers such as Orlistat® deplete the body of the essential fats it needs for every cell, by preventing their absorption. Thus they also prevent the absorption of fat soluble vitamins, such as vitamins A, D, E, and K. Further, fat-blockers do not prevent excess carbohydrates from being turned into and stored in the body as fat. Given that most people consume too many carbohydrates for their activity level, this class of weight-loss drugs fails to address part of the root problem of most overweight people's diet. So, despite blocking the absorption of fat, they will still potentially store fat where they do not want to. In addition, these fat-blockers cause an essential fatty acid deficiency in the process.

Weight-loss surgery

Surgery is an option for patients with extreme obesity. Weight loss surgery provides medically significant sustained weight loss for more than five years in most patients. Although there are risks associated with surgery, it is not yet known whether these risks are greater in the long term than those of any other form of treatment. Surgery is an option for well-informed and motivated patients who have clinically severe obesity (BMI ≥ 40) or a (BMI ≥ 35) and serious comorbid conditions. (The term "clinically severe obesity" is preferred to the once commonly used term "morbid obesity.") Surgical patients should be monitored for complications and lifestyle adjustments throughout their lives.

[JA] Although practitioners of Chinese medicine do not administer pharmacotherapy or perform surgery, I have included this information because we can, nevertheless, take an active part in weight loss maintenance when these therapies have been used. Furthermore, some of our patients will be advised by a medical doctor to consider these therapies and will ask our advice. Therefore, we should know all we can about when pharmacotherapy or surgery is or is not clinically indicated. This knowledge allows us to engage in an informed, professional discussion with the patient about the short and long-term effectiveness of such treatments along with non-invasive techniques for weight maintenance. This knowledge also allows us to recognize patients for whom these treatments would be contraindicated, such as patients who do not suffer from severe obesity (BMI ≥ 40) or a (BMI ≥ 35) and serious comorbid conditions or other circumstances. For example, take a female patient who plans to have children. We might ask her to consider avoiding bariatric surgery because she could risk nutrient deficiency in the developing baby. Bariatric surgery reduces the stomach size, thus significantly reducing the amount of nutrients a woman can absorb. This thus reduces the nourishment available for the developing baby. Nutrient deficiencies in pregnant mothers can result in serious adverse effects on the developing baby. Simply taking prenatal vitamins does not solve this problem because such vitamins are meant as supplements to pregnant mothers. They are not meant as a replacement for nutrients derived from food. For these reasons, Chinese medicine practitioners should stay advised of all treatments and possible adverse effects.

Special Situations

Involve other health professionals when possible, especially for special situations. Although research regarding obesity treatment in older people is not abundant, age should not preclude therapy for obesity. In people who smoke, the risk of weight gain is often a barrier to smoking cessation. In these patients, cessation of smoking should be encouraged first, and weight loss therapy should be an additional goal. A weight loss and maintenance program can be conducted by a practitioner without specialization in weight loss so long as that person has the requisite interest and knowledge. However, a variety of practitioners with special skills are available and may be enlisted to assist in the development of a program.

[JA] Chinese medical practitioners can play a crucial role in the treatment of overweight and obesity. Practitioners of Chinese medicine treat with acupuncture, Chinese herbs, diet therapy, and behavioral change. Many of us have training in exercise therapy, tai chi, qigong, or yoga. Many have training in smoking cessation, mindfulness-based stress reduction techniques, meditation, and breath-work among many other skills. Our holistic medicine fits within the NIH standards for practice, and most of the NIH standards of practice fit within the holistic treatment paradigm of traditional Chinese medicine.

Contraindications for Weight Loss Treatment

- Pregnant and nursing mothers.

- Anorexic and bulimic patients.

- Patients being treated for severe depression.

(However, weight maintenance programs may be indicated in these cases.)

The Chinese Medical Causes & Mechanisms of Being Overweight

3

In order to understand how Chinese medicine treats overweight and obesity, one must first understand what fat is and how it is produced according to the theories of Chinese medicine. To begin with, the concept of health within Chinese medicine is based on the Confucian doctrine of the meaning (*zhong yong* 中用). This means

> In terms of overweight, everyone needs to have a moderate amount of adipose tissue. Conversely, either too much or too little adipose tissue results in disease.

that nothing is good or bad in and of itself as long as it is within normal parameters—neither too much or too little depending on the situation. In terms of overweight, everyone needs to have a moderate amount of adipose tissue. Fat accumulates in the adipose tissue, but either too much or too little adipose tissue results in disease. If one is overweight, the disease is simply called fatness (*fei pang* 肥膀) in Chinese, while if one is too thin, the disease is called emaciation (*xiao shou* 消瘦). Both fatness and emaciation are disease categories in traditional Chinese medicine. Also in Chinese medicine, a healthy, moderate amount of adipose tissue is referred to as flesh (*rou*肉), and flesh is always seen as something positive. This flesh gives the body its rounded appearance, and, when combined with muscle (*ji* 肌, as in *ji rou* 肌肉), it is what gives the body its strength and ability to move in space. This rounded appearance is a result of the construction and nourishment provided by the spleen from the finest essence of food and drink taken in by the stomach. Fat (*fei* 肥) , on the other hand, always refers to an excess. Unlike flesh, the concept of fat is never seen as something healthy. In Chinese medicine, fat is nothing other than a pathological accumulation of phlegm, dampness, and turbidity. For instance, Dr. Sun Li says in an article published on the acupuncture treatment of simple obesity in 2004, fat is categorized as a species of "heavy phlegm, turbidity, and dampness." It is formed due to non-transformation of righteous fluids and humors. These collect and accumulate and produce fat. Below, we look at the engenderment of each of these three evils, beginning with turbidity.

Turbidity & the spleen

As soon as a Chinese medical practitioner says the word turbidity (*zhuo* 浊), other Chinese medical practitioners know we are mainly talking about the functions of the spleen and stomach as defined by Chinese medicine. The spleen and stomach are the two main organs which control digestion, and they work in a coordinated and interdependent way. The stomach receives food and drink which it "rottens and ripens." The spleen then upbears the clear (*qing* 清) part of this "mash" to the lungs and heart in order for it to be transformed into qi and blood respectively. The stomach downbears the turbid part of this mash to the intestines and bladder for eventual discharge from the body as feces and urine. This upbearing of the clear and downbearing of the turbid are interdependent. The turbid can only be downborne if the clear is upborne and vice versa. Further, the stomach qi, that which empowers the stomach's function, comes from the spleen. What this means is that accumulation of turbidity is mainly due to spleen dysfunction in Chinese medicine.

Dampness & the spleen

Dampness (*shi* 湿) in Chinese medicine refers to water fluids (*shui ye* 水液) which have not been transformed and have ceased to move, and it is the spleen which governs movement and transformation of water fluids. Further, it is specifically the spleen qi which empowers this movement and transformation. Therefore, anything which obstructs the function of the spleen qi or causes it to decrease in amount may result in the accumulation of dampness.

Phlegm & the spleen

Phlegm (*tan* 痰) in Chinese medicine is nothing other than congealed dampness. Dampness may congeal due to cold, heat, or simply because it has collected and endured for a long period of time. Because phlegm is nothing other than congealed dampness, dampness is nothing other than collected water fluids, and the spleen governs the movement and transformation of water fluids, it is commonly said that, "The spleen is the root of phlegm engenderment." Clinically, this means that there is some element of spleen dysfunction in all cases of overweight and obesity.

What causes spleen dysfunction? The answers are vacuity and encumbrance. Spleen qi may be too vacuous and weak to perform its functions of moving and transforming. The things that Chinese medical theory says can cause spleen qi vacuity are insufficient exercise, too much thinking and worry, taxation fatigue, aging, chronic disease, over or inappropriate use of certain types of medicinals, and unregulated eating and drinking. In particular, this latter means eating too much sugar and sweets, too much fatty food, too many foods which strongly engender fluids, and eating too much raw (*sheng* 生 , uncooked) and chilled (*leng* 冷) foods. Spleen encumbrance means that the function of the spleen qi is inhibited by some evil qi. Most typically this is dampness since "the spleen is averse to dampness." This dampness may be either externally contracted, such as by living in a damp environment, or may be internally engendered, such as by eating too many foods which strongly engender fluids. However, the spleen qi may also be hindered and encumbered by eating too much food in general and eating too much hard-to-digest food in particular. Both of these may cause food stagnation which damages the spleen.

Other viscera & bowels involved in overweight & obesity

There are three viscera and two bowels including the spleen that are involved in being overweight. When it comes to the control over water fluids in the body, the lungs and kidneys also play an important role. Together, the lungs, spleen, and kidneys are the three viscera which govern water fluids in the body. Because each is located in one of the three burners, upper, middle, and lower respectively, it is also said that the triple burner governs the water passageways.

The kidneys

The kidneys are probably the next most important of the above three viscera in the control of water fluids in the body. In Chinese medicine just as in Western medicine, the kidneys are in charge of creating and discharging urine, and the urine is seen as a turbid fluid. Thus the kidneys directly influence the amount of turbid fluids accumulated within the body. However, the function of the kidneys and spleen are interdependent. The kidneys are the former heaven root, the spleen is the latter heaven root, and former and latter heavens mutually support and promote each other. In terms of being overweight, this primarily means that spleen yang is rooted in kidney yang. If, for any reason, the spleen qi and yang become vacuous and weak, eventually so will kidney qi and yang and vice versa. In particular, the spleen becomes vacuous and weak due to aging in the mid-30s and 40s, and this leads to kidney

vacuity in the late 40s and 50s. In this case, there is a spleen-kidney dual
vacuity, and the presence of this dual vacuity is closely related to the typical
gain in weight of the late middle-aged and young elderly. In Chinese medicine, the most basic treatment principle for dealing with phlegm is to transform phlegm (*hua tan* 化痰), but the word "transform" is also the word—to
melt—in Chinese. Thus the transformation of phlegm is dependent on the
warm yang qi of the spleen and kidneys in order to accomplish that "melt-
ing."

What are the things that can make kidney yang vacuous and insufficient?
The first is aging. The kidneys become vacuous and insufficient in most people by at least the age of 60 and often 10 years before that, especially in
females. Other things that can cause kidney vacuity are enduring disease, certain types of medicinals, all recreational drugs, and all types of extreme physical and mental activity.

The lungs

The lungs are said to be "the upper source of water in the body." It is the lung
qi which diffuses the fluids upborne by the spleen from the digestate. In other
words, it is the lung qi which provides the power of movement for water fluids to flow through the channels and vessels of the body. This is based on the
statement, "The qi moves water fluids. If the qi moves, fluids move. If the qi
stops, fluids stop." If this lung qi is either insufficient in amount or its diffusion and downbearing are inhibited by some evil qi, water fluids will not
move downward. Instead they will stop and collect and transform into dampness. If this dampness lingers and endures, it will eventually congeal into
phlegm. Because the lung qi comes from the spleen qi, spleen qi vacuity may
and often does evolve into lung-spleen qi vacuity. In that case, the creation of
phlegm dampness is all the more likely.

What causes lung qi vacuity? Excessive speaking (including chanting and
singing), spleen qi vacuity as noted above, tobacco smoking, and enduring
disease are the main causes of lung qi vacuity. Evil qi causing inhibition of
the diffusion and downbearing of the lung qi may be due to external con-
traction of wind, cold, heat, and dryness evils, internally engendered heat
floating upward, yin vacuity of the lungs, kidneys, and/or stomach, and
phlegm dampness accumulated in the lungs. While the lungs rarely play a
lead role in the creation of excessive adipose tissue, they may definitely play a
contributory role, especially once the patient has become overweight.

The liver

The liver, on the other hand, typically does play a major role in the creation of phlegm, dampness, and turbidity and, therefore, in being overweight. The liver is responsible for maintaining the free flow of the qi mechanism. This means two things. First it means that the liver maintains the free flow of the qi throughout the entire body. If, for any reason, the liver qi becomes depressed and bound, the qi will fail to move water fluids. If these water fluids stop and collect, we have already seen how they first transform into evil dampness and eventually congeal into phlegm. However, the qi mechanism also describes the upbearing of the clear by the spleen and the downbearing of the turbid by the stomach, and the liver has a very close relationship with both the spleen and stomach. In fact, this relationship is so close that it is said, "Liver disease is spleen disease," and, "If the liver is diseased, first treat the spleen." If the liver becomes depressed and the qi becomes stagnant, the qi mechanism becomes inhibited and loses its free flow. The spleen qi fails to upbear the clear and the stomach then fails to downbear the turbid. Thus clear and turbid are not separated and turbidity accumulates within the body. Further, when the liver assails the spleen, the spleen qi becomes vacuous and weak. It then fails to govern the movement and transformation of water fluids. Dampness is engendered and dampness over time leads to the creation of phlegm.

> "If the liver is diseased, first treat the spleen."

Unfortunately, dampness and phlegm may also cause or aggravate liver depression. Because qi and fluids move together, if dampness or phlegm are created in the body, they will hinder and obstruct the free flow of the qi. This then will damage and depress the liver, leading to qi stagnation which will then lead to even more dampness and phlegm. This creates a mutually reinforcing loop where liver depression causes spleen vacuity and phlegm dampness but spleen vacuity and phlegm dampness create more liver depression qi stagnation.

What causes liver depression? Unfulfilled desires and great anger are the two main psychological causes of liver depression. However, there are a number of physiological causes which can also cause or aggravate liver depression. These include blood vacuity due to menstruation, gestation, and/or lactation, yin vacuity and/or yang vacuity due to aging, or the enduring existence of any other evil qi in the body, whether externally contracted or internally engendered. This especially includes wind, cold, dampness, phlegm, food stagnation, and blood stasis.

The stomach

As we have seen above, if the spleen qi fails to empower the stomach, the stomach may fail to downbear turbidity and turbidity may accumulate. While this turbidity remains within the stomach, it is called food stagnation. Unfortunately, this food stagnation may damage the spleen leading to even more spleen vacuity. When this happens, yet another mutually reinforcing loop is created. However, the stomach plays yet another role in the internal engenderment of phlegm and dampness and thus excessive adipose tissue. The spleen-stomach qi is directly responsible for the appetite. When the spleen and stomach qi are both vacuous and weak, the appetite is poor. However, when the stomach qi is exuberant, the appetite is normal or strong *even when the spleen qi is vacuous and weak.* Worse yet, when the stomach qi is hot, the appetite is excessive or even ravenous no matter if the spleen is vacuous. Qi promotes function, and the function of the stomach is to downbear the turbid, but heat is nothing other than a lot of qi. This means that, if the stomach becomes hot, it also hyperfunctions, and hyperfunction of the stomach means rapid emptying. This leads to rapid hungering and excessive appetite. Unfortunately, when the spleen becomes vacuous and weak with aging in middle or late middle age, the stomach often remains healthily strong or even pathologically hot. Thus the person overeats while the spleen is not able to separate clear from turbid, phlegm and dampness are engendered internally, and the person gains weight. When it comes to central obesity (excess weight carried in the abdomen and waist area), there is almost always a hot stomach (and possibly intestines) no matter what else is also going on.

The large intestine

Most Chinese medical textbooks do not discuss the role of the large intestine in being overweight or obese. Nevertheless, there is such a role. In Chinese medicine, the stomach and large intestine are closely related. Together, the stomach and large intestine channels form the yang ming. If, for any reason, the stomach is hot, it may cause heat in the large intestine as well. If this heat damages intestinal fluids, it may lead to constipation, and, if there is constipation, turbidity is not efficiently discharged from the body. On the other hand, large intestine heat will tend to aggravate stomach heat, making the stomach even hotter. Therefore, the patient may eat or at least be tempted to eat even more. This means that the free flow of the large intestine is directly related to the accumulation of turbidity in the body and the amount of heat in the stomach. Further, if there is constipation, there is non-free flow of the large intestine qi. Because the liver qi governs the coursing and discharge of the qi of the entire body, large intestine qi stagnation may cause or aggravate liver depression qi stagnation, and we have seen how liver depression can lead to phlegm dampness. While dysfunction of the large intestine rarely causes overweight by itself, it can and often does complicate other disease mechanisms more directly involved in the accumulation of phlegm, dampness, and turbidity within the body.

Blood stasis

Blood stasis (*xue yu* 血瘀) is yet another, although frequently overlooked, factor in the development of excessive adipose tissue. In Chinese medicine, blood and fluids move together. Static blood is dry, dead, unmoving blood. If blood stasis is created due to any reason, this static blood will hinder the free flow of water fluids. Instead, these water fluids will stop and collect and transform into dampness. If the dampness remains long enough, dampness will congeal into phlegm. Therefore, blood stasis may cause phlegm dampness to accumulate in the body. On the other hand, phlegm and dampness may both hinder and obstruct the free flow of blood, eventually causing blood stasis. What this means is that most patients who are overweight suffer from some element of blood stasis over time. While blood stasis may not be the initiating factor in becoming overweight, once created, it does aggravate the presence of phlegm dampness and thus prevents that weight from being shed. Besides the presence of phlegm dampness, other important causes of blood stasis include liver depression qi stagnation, chronic disease, and aging.

Yin & yang

Yin and yang are the two main overarching principles of Chinese medicine. When all is said and done, phlegm, dampness, and turbidity are all yin evils. Their accumulation means that, at least where the excessive adipose tissue exists, there is insufficient yang qi to move and transform that phlegm and dampness. Such yang qi insufficiency may be due to a true systemic yang qi insufficiency (primarily of the spleen and kidneys) or it may be due to a local blockage by some evil qi, such as phlegm, dampness, food stagnation, qi stagnation, and/or blood stasis. It is also possible and commonly seen in clinical practice that the spleen and kidneys are vacuous and weak while the stomach is hot and hyperactive. In this case, there is a mixed yin and yang situation. And finally, it must be mentioned that people are born with inherent differences in their yin and yang and the strengths and weaknesses of individual organs. Therefore, Chinese medicine does recognize that some people are constitutionally prone to being overweight. This is referred to as "habitual bodily phlegm dampness" in Chinese medicine.

The Treatment of Overweight & Obesity with Chinese Medicine

4

The traditional Chinese medical approach to weight loss is to treat each patient's individually manifesting disease mechanisms resulting in the accumulation of phlegm, dampness, and turbidity, and that means treating based on the patient's personally presenting patterns. Within professional Chinese medicine, there is no one-size-fits-all treatment. In clinical practice, we first identify the patient's unique Chinese medical patterns using inquiry and examination and then base the treatment upon that pattern discrimination using the treatment principles as the bridge between these two. In addition, overweight patients typically present with other disease diagnoses. Some other conditions commonly associated with obesity are high cholesterol, diabetes, hypertension, osteoarthritis, back or knee pain, depression, and heart disease. Depending on the condition and whether or not it shares one or more disease mechanisms with the overweight, we may also (and usually) choose to treat these as well. When such comorbidities are taken into account, treatment tends to be even more individualized.

In general, the following are the usual steps in treating overweight with Chinese medicine:

- Differentiate the pattern(s)
- State the treatment principles for that/those pattern(s)
- Erect a treatment plan using acupuncture and/or Chinese herbal medicine and diet and lifestyle recommendations based upon those treatment principles
- Adjust the pattern differentiation and treatment plan according to the patient's changes over the course of treatment

Treatment based on pattern discrimination

The following are the main patterns of overweight and obesity recognized today within professional Chinese medicine. For didactic purposes, they are presented as individual, discrete patterns. However, in real life, patients tend to present with multi-pattern combinations. Therefore, the treatment protocols under each pattern are given as examples only and will typically need to be modified with additions and subtractions.

I. Stomach heat & damp blockage (*wei re shi bi,* 胃热湿闭)

Signs & symptoms: Obesity, head distention, dizziness, rapid hungering after eating, heaviness of the limbs which caused them to be indolent, thirst, a predilection for drinking, constipation, a red tongue with slimy, slightly yellow fur, and a slippery, slightly rapid pulse

Note: In this case, being overweight is due to overeating in turn due to stomach heat. The stomach takes in more food and drink than the spleen can move and transform. The excess then becomes dampness and phlegm.

Treatment principles: Clear heat and eliminate dampness

Acupuncture-moxibustion:
Nei Ting (St 44)
Jie Xi (St 41)
Yin Ling Quan (Sp 9)
Feng Long (St 40)
Zhong Wan (CV 12)
Tian Shu (St 25)
Da Chang Shu (Bl 25)

Formula explanation: *Nei Ting* and *Jie Xi* clear heat from the stomach. *Yin Ling Quan* seeps dampness. *Zhong Wan* and *Feng Long* transform phlegm. *Tian Shu* and *Da Chang Shu* free the flow of the stools, clear and precipitate.

Additions & subtractions: For head distention and dizziness, add *Tai Yang* (M-HN-9) and *Feng Chi* (GB 20). For thirst, add *Cheng Jiang* (CV 24) and *Zhao Hai* (Ki 6). For constipation, add *Zhi Gou* (TB 6) and *Zhao Hai*.

Chinese herbal formula: *Fang Feng Tong Sheng Tang* (Ledebouriella Sagely Free the Flow Decoction)

Ingredients:
Shi Gao (Gypsum Fibrosum), 12g
Hua Shi (Talcum), 12g
Fang Feng (Radix Ledebouriella), 9g
Jing Jie Sui (Herba Schizonepetae), 9g
Zhi Zi (Fructus Gardeniae), 9g
Lian Qiao (Fructus Forsythiae), 9g
Huang Qin (Radix Scutellariae), 9g
Jie Geng (Radix Platycodi), 9g
Bai Zhu (Radix Atractylodis Macrocephalae), 9g
Bai Shao (Radix Alba Paeoniae), 9g
Dang Gui (Radix Angelicae Sinensis), 9g
Chuan Xiong (Radix Chuanxiong), 3-6g
Ma Huang (Herba Ephedrae), 3-6g
Bo He (Herba Menthae Haplocalycis), 3-6g
Da Huang (Radix Et Rhizoma Rhei), 3-6g
Mang Xiao (Natri Sulfas), 3-6g
Gan Cao (Radix Glycyrrhizae), 3-6g
Sheng Jiang (uncooked Rhizoma Zingiberis), 2-3 slices

Formula explanation: *Shi Gao, Hua Shi, Zhi Zi, Lian Qiao, Huang Qin, Jing Jie Sui, Bo He, Da Huang,* and *Mang Xiao* all clear heat. *Hua Shi* also seeps dampness, while *Bo He* and *Jing Jie Sui* resolve the exterior and move and rectify the qi. *Ma Huang* strongly resolves the exterior. It, along with *Jing Jie Sui* and *Bo He*, are windy, acrid medicinals which upbear and out-thrust yang. From a Western biomedical point of view, *Ma Huang* stimulates and increases the basal metabolic rate. *Da Huang* and *Mang Xiao* also discharge heat, free the flow of the stools, and relieve constipation. *Bai Zhu* fortifies the spleen and dries dampness. *Jie Geng* transforms phlegm and also guides the other medicinals to the upper half of the body. Thus this formula is targeted to treat central obesity. *Bai Shao, Dang Gui,* and *Chuan Xiong* nourish and quicken the blood. By nourishing the blood, they help prevent the attacking and draining medicinals from damaging the righteous. By quickening the blood, they help prevent phlegm and dampness from engendering stasis. *Sheng Jiang* aids *Jie Geng* in transforming phlegm. It also eliminates dampness and harmonizes the stomach. Along with *Gan Cao*, it also harmonizes and regulates all the other medicinals in the formula. With the exception of *Bai Zhu, Dang Gui,* and *Bai Shao,* all the ingredients in this formula are draining, and this formula as a whole is strongly attacking and draining. It should only be used in patients with a replete constitution.

Additions & subtractions: If there is no constipation, delete *Da Huang* and *Mang Xiao* or use only with care.

Ready-made Chinese medicines: *Fang Feng Tong Sheng Wan* (Ledebouirella Sagely Free the Flow Pills). Note that the Plum Flower version of this formula does not include *Ma Huang* which has been banned by the U.S. FDA from inclusion in dietary supplements.

Diet & lifestyle: Cut back on the amounts of spicy, peppery, hot foods and fried and fatty foods. Also cut back on alcohol consumption. All these things can make the stomach hotter and, therefore, increase the appetite. In addition, fatty, oily foods also strongly engender fluids which may easily be transformed into phlegm dampness. This includes dairy products such as milk, cheese, cream, and butter. Eat more slowly and chew more thoroughly. This can also help reduce the stomach's hyperfunctioning. In particular, eat more cool and cold foods as described by Chinese medicine. This means such foods as lettuce, celery, cucumbers, zucchini, and bitter melon. The Chinese medical natures (*i.e.*, temperatures) of many commonly eaten foods are found in Appendix B in the back of this book.

2. Food stagnation with constipation (*shi zhi bian bi*, 食滞便秘)

Signs & symptoms: Obesity with abdominal distention and oppression, belching and sour eructation, bad breath, constipation, thick, slimy tongue fur, and a slippery pulse

Note: Food stagnation with or without constipation is rarely the sole disease mechanism of overweight. However, food stagnation complicates many other patterns.

Treatment principles: Disperse food and abduct stagnation, free the flow of the stools and relieve constipation

Acupuncture-moxibustion:
Nei Ting (St 44)
Shang Wan (CV 10)
Zhong Wan (CV 12)
Xia Wan (CV 13)
Liang Men (St 21)
Tian Shu (St 25)
Da Chang Shu (Bl 25)

Formula explanation: *Nei Ting* drains repletions from the stomach. When used together, *Shang Wan, Zhong Wan*, and *Xia Wan* strongly disinhibit the qi mechanism, promoting the upbearing of the clear and the downbearing of the turbid. *Liang Men* abducts foods and disperses stagnation. *Tian Shu* and *Da Chang Shu* free the flow of the stools and relieve constipation.

Additions & subtractions: If there is constipation, add *Zhi Gou* (TB 6) and *Zhao Hai* (Ki 6). If there is nausea, add *Nei Guan* (Per 6) and *Zu San Li* (St 36). To transform phlegm and eliminate dampness more, add *Feng Long* (St 40).

Chinese herbal formula: *Xiao Cheng Qi Tang* (Minor Order the Qi Decoction) plus *Bao He Wan* (Protect Harmony Pills) with additions and subtractions:

Ingredients:
Hou Po (Cortex Magnoliae Officinalis), 9g
Zhi Shi (Fructus Immaturus Aurantii), 9g
Bing Lang (Semen Arecae), 9g
Shan Zha (Fructus Crataegi), 9g
Ban Xia (Rhizoma Pinelliae), 9g
Shen Qu (Massa Medica Fermentata), 9g
Lai Fu Zi (Semen Raphani), 9g
Da Huang (Radix Et Rhizoma Rhei), 3-6g

Formula explanation: Within this formula, *Shan Zha, Shen Qu*, and *Lai Fu Zi* abduct stagnation and disperse food. *Hou Po, Zhi Shi*, and *Ban Xia* harmonize the stomach, transform phlegm, and downbear turbidity. *Bing Lang* moves the qi downward and seeps dampness. *Da Huang* frees the flow of the stools and relieves constipation.

Additions & subtractions: For more prominent constipation, add *Mang Xiao* (Natri Sulfas), 3-6g. For more marked dampness and phlegm, add *Fu Ling* (Poria), 9-12g, and *Chen Pi* (Pericarpium Citri Reticulatae), 6-9g.

For a patient with a replete constitution with primarily stomach heat and constipation, consider *Da Cheng Qi Tang* (Major Order the Qi Decoction) at least until the constipation is resolved:

Hou Po (Cortex Magnoliae), 12g
Zhi Shi (Fructus Immaturus Aurantii), 6-9g
Da Huang (Radix Et Rhizoma Rhei*), 6-9g
Mang Xiao (Natri Sulfas), 3-6g

Formula explanation: All four ingredients in this formula free the flow of the stools, drain the stomach and intestines. *Da Huang* and *Mang Xiao* clear heat from the stomach and intestines and discharge turbidity. *Zhi Shi* also strongly moves the qi and transforms phlegm. *Hou Po* moves the qi in the middle and disperses stagnation, dries dampness and transforms phlegm.

Ready-made Chinese medicines: *Tao Ren Wan* (Persica Seed Pills) a.k.a. *Run Chang Wan* (Moisten the Intestine Pills) plus *Bao He Wan* (Protect Harmony Pills)

Diet & lifestyle: Cut back on the amount of food eaten at any one time and do not eat until absolutely full. Also cut back on foods which are hard-to-digest, such as crusty, hard breads, beef jerky, nuts, etc. These foods tend to aggravate food stagnation. For food stagnation, add papaya, pineapple, malt, and/or digestive enzymes to aid digestion. For constipation, consider adding some figs or prunes to one's diet and maybe do regular abdominal massage. Other options for constipation include eating apples or drinking aloe vera juice. In general, be sure to eat plenty of fiber. For instructions on how to do abdominal massage, see below. Other suggestions for dealing with food stagnation are to take a 20 minute walk after eating and to wait at least 30 minutes before lying down after eating.

Abdominal Massage Instructions for Patients

Be sure to administer this massage to patients as you instruct them how to self-administer. Refer to the following illustration.

1. Sit up in a comfortable chair.
2. With two of your right fingers, press into your right hip on the front of the pelvis. (A)
3. With two left fingers, touch your belly button. (B)
4. With your two left fingers, trace an imaginary line from your belly button to your right hip bone stopping about two-thirds of the way toward the hip point. This is the area of the illiocecal valve, the valve that allows food through the small intestine (from the stomach) into the large intestine.
5. Gently press the two left fingers into the area of the illiocecal valve which may feel tender. Release your right fingers from the hip point.
6. With your left fingers pressed into the spot on your abdomen, massage the area with a back and forth motion from the belly button to the hip point and back again. Do this for 1-2 minutes. This massage will help to open the illiocecal valve, which sometimes gets stuck, allowing backed up waste to move out of the stomach, into the small intestine, through the valve, into the large intestine and eventually out of the body.

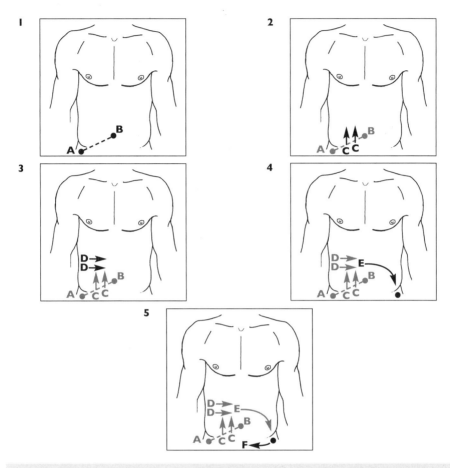

7. When you have finished massaging the valve, relax your fingers. Now use flat fingers from both hands and slowly massage in both a circular and upward motion tracing the large intestine up the abdomen toward the ribcage. (C)

8. Once you reach the ribcage, massage across the abdomen toward the left. The large intestine curves an inch or so below your right ribcage. (D) Blockages in any area of the intestine usually feel like a mass and are sometimes tender to the touch. If there is blockage in the curve, massage the blockage by following the curve of the intestine. Massage this area even if there is not a blockage. (E)

9. When you reach the left ribcage, massage in circles down and around the curve, then massage in downward circles toward the left hip point.

10. When you reach the left hip point, massage in a clockwise manner around and down the curve toward the right hip. (F)

11. Continue massaging your large intestine in this clockwise manner for

continued

about five to ten minutes. You can bring the clockwise movement closer toward the navel each time you massage around the abdomen.

12. Always end the massage in the lower abdomen a couple of inches below the navel.

Administer this massage to your illiocecal valve and large intestine daily for at least five minutes per day. Wait at least 30 minutes after eating before administering abdominal massage. This massage can be performed in the bathroom to promote an immediate bowel movement for patients who have stools that are hard to move.

3. Phlegm dampness brewing internally (*tan shi nei yun*, 痰湿内蕴)

Signs & symptoms: Obesity, a predilection for sweet, fatty foods and dairy products or alcohol, chest and stomach glomus and oppression, nausea, profuse phlegm, dizziness, heart palpitations, heavy, fatigued limbs, somnolence, an enlarged tongue with thick, slimy fur, and a bowstring, slippery, forceful pulse

Note: Although the name of this pattern contains no reference to food stagnation, its treatments do address this cofactor.

Treatment principles: Transform phlegm and dry dampness, abduct accumulation and disperse food

Acupuncture-moxibustion:
Yin Ling Quan (Sp 9)
San Yin Jiao (St 6)
Zu San Li (St 36)
Feng Long (St 40)
Xia Wan (CV 10)
Shui Fen (CV 9)

Formula explanation: Within this formula, *Yin Ling Quan*, *San Yin Jiao*, and *Shui Fen* eliminate dampness via disinhibiting urination. *Zu San Li* and *Xia Wan* downbear turbidity, abduct accumulation, and disperse food. In addition, *Zu San Li* and *San Yin Jiao*, by fortifying the spleen, help to dry damp ness via transformation. *Feng Long* specifically transforms phlegm.

Additions & subtractions: For profuse sweating, add *He Gu* (LI 4) and *Fu Liu* (Ki 7). For somnolence and disliking movement, moxa *San Jiao Shu* (Bl 22).

Chinese herbal formula: Modified *Er Chen Tang* (Two Aged [Ingredients] Decoction) plus *Ping Wei San* (Level [*i.e.*, Calm] the Stomach Powder)

Ingredients:
Ban Xia (Rhizoma Pinelliae), 9g
Chen Pi (Pericarpium Citri Reticulatae), 9g
Fu Ling (Poria), 9g
Hou Po (Cortex Magnoliae), 9g
Bai Zhu (Rhizoma Atractylodis Macrocephalae), 9g
Shan Zha (Fructus Crataegi), 9g
Lai Fu Zi (Semen Raphani), 9g
He Ye (Folium Nelumbinis), 9g
Cang Zhu (Rhizoma Atractylodis), 6g
Zhi Ke (Fructus Aurantii), 6g
mix-fried *Gan Cao* (Radix Glycyrrhizae), 3g

Formula explanation: *Ban Xia, Fu Ling, Hou Po, Chen Pi*, and *Zhi Ke* transform phlegm and eliminate dampness. They also harmonize the stomach and downbear turbidity. *Bai Zhu, Cang Zhu, Fu Ling, Lian Zi*, and mix-fried *Gan Cao* fortify the spleen and, thereby, eliminate dampness. In particular, *Bai Zhu* fortifies the spleen and transforms dampness, while *Cang Zhu* dries dampness and fortifies the spleen. *Shan Zha* and *Lai Fu Zi* abduct stagnation and disperse food. In addition, *Bai Zhu, Cang Zhu*, and *He Ye* are all empirically known to lower serum glucose levels, while *Shan Zha* is known to reduce serum lipids.

Additions & subtractions: For fear of cold, add *Gan Jiang* (dry Rhizoma Zingiberis), 6g, and *Gui Zhi* (Ramulus Cinnamomi), 9g. For aversion to heat and yellow phlegm, subtract *Cang Zhu* and add *Zhu Ru* (Caulis Bambusae In Taeniis), 9g, *Huang Qin* (Radix Scutellariae), 6g, and *Hua Shi* (Talcum), 6g. For inhibited urination, add *Ze Xie* (Rhizoma Alismatis), 9g, and *Han Fang Ji* (Radix Stephaniae Tetrandrae), 9g. For constipation, add *Fan Xie Ye* (Folium Sennae), 3-9g. For somnolence, add *Shi Chang Pu* (Rhizoma Acori Tatarinowii), 9g.

Ready-made Chinese medicines: *Er Chen Wan* (Two Aged [Ingredients] Pills) plus *Bao He Wan* (Protect Harmony Pills)

Diet & lifestyle: Do not eat too many fats and oils, including as stated above, diary products. These foods strongly engender fluids which may transform into phlegm and dampness. Do not eat many sugars and sweets. These foods damage the spleen and also engender fluids. Remember, "The spleen is the root of phlegm engenderment." Get more exercise. The qi moves water fluids and exercise moves the qi. If the qi moves, water fluids move. Consider radiant heat saunas to also melt fat, sweat more, and increase the flow of qi.

4. Spleen qi vacuity weakness (*pi wei xu ruo*, 脾胃虚弱)

Signs & symptoms: Obesity with a long history of bad dietary habits, fatigue, lack of strength, laziness to speak, fatigued spirit, a puffy face, a poor appetite (as long as the stomach is not also hot), abdominal fullness after eating, loose stools, possible clear, thin vaginal discharge, possible bland taste in the mouth, a pale tongue with teeth-marks on its edges and thin, white fur, and a fine, forceless pulse

Treatment principles: Fortify the spleen, supplement the qi, disinhibit urination and seep dampness

Acupuncture-moxibustion:
Pi Shu (Bl 20)
Wei Shu (Bl 23)
Zu San Li (St 36)
San Yin Jiao (Sp 6)
Zhong Wan (CV 12)

Formula explanation: *Pi Shu, Wei Shu, San Yin Jiao, Zhong Wan*, and *Zu San Li* all fortify the spleen and supplement the qi.

Additions & subtractions: For spleen yang vacuity, add moxibustion at *Pi Shu, Wei Shu, Zhong Wan*, and *Zu San Li*. In addition, a TDP lamp may be used on the upper abdomen and lower thorax on the back.

Chinese herbal formula: Modified *Liu Jun Zi Tang* (Six Gentlemen Decoction) plus *Fang Ji Huang Qi Tang* (Stephania & Astragalus Decoction)

Ingredients:
Huang Qi (Radix Astragali), 15g
Han Fang Ji (Radix Stephaniae Tetrandrae), 12g
Dang Shen (Radix Codonopsis), 9g
Bai Zhu (Rhizoma Atractylodis Macrocephalae), 9g
Fu Ling (Poria), 9g
Ban Xia (Rhizoma Pinelliae), 9g
Shan Zha (Fructus Crataegi), 9g

Chen Pi (Pericarpium Citri Reticulatae), 6g
mix-fried *Gan Cao* (Radix Glycyrrhizae), 3g

Formula explanation: *Huang Qi, Dang Shen, Bai Zhu, Fu Ling,* and mix-fried *Gan Cao* fortify the spleen and supplement the qi. *Han Fan Ji* and *Fu Ling* seep dampness and disperse swelling. *Ban Xia* and *Chen Pi,* transform phlegm, eliminate dampness, and downbear turbidity. *Shan Zha* abducts stagnation and disperses food. *Han Fang Ji* is a common ingredient in Chinese weight loss formulas. However, because it is commonly substituted by Aristolochia species containing the nephrotoxin aristolochic acid, it should only be used if one can guarantee that it is indeed Radix Stephaniae Tetrandrae.

Additions & subtractions: For stomach and abdominal fullness and distention, add *Mu Xiang* (Radix Auklandiae), 6g, *Sha Ren* (Fructus Amomi), 6g, and *He Ye* (Folium Nelumbinis), 9g. For inhibited urination, add *Ze Xie* (Rhizoma Alismatis), 9g.

For diarrhea with sliminess in the mouth, replace *Liu Jun Zi Tang* plus *Fang Ji Huang Qi Tang* with modified *Shen Ling Bai Zhu San* (Ginseng, Poria & Atractylodes Powder):

Yi Yi Ren (Semen Coicis), 15g
Bai Zhu (Rhizoma Atractylodis Macrocephalae), 12g
Bai Bian Dou (Semen Dolichoris), 9g
Shan Yao (Radix Dioscoreae), 9g
Fu Ling (Poria), 9g
Dang Shen (Radix Codonopsis), 9g
Shan Zha (Fructus Crataegi), 9g
He Ye (Folium Nelumbinis), 9g
Lian Zi (Semen Nelumbinis), 6g
mix-fried *Gan Cao* (Radix Glycyrrhizae), 6g

Formula explanation: *Yi Yi Ren, Bai Zhu, Bai Bian Dou, Shan Yao, Fu Ling, Lian Zi,* and mix-fried *Gan Cao* all fortify the spleen and supplement the qi. *Shan Yao, Bai Bian Dou,* and *Lian Zi* empirically stop diarrhea. *Yi Yi Ren, Bai Zhu, Bai Bian Dou,* and *Fu Ling* eliminate dampness by both transforming and seeping it. *Shan Zha* abducts stagnation and disperses food. *He Ye* clears heat from the stomach and empirically reduces fat and lowers blood sugar.

For spleen qi vacuity complicated by dampness and turbidity, qi and food stagnation, and blood stasis, consider using *Wu Long Jiang Zhi Tang* (Oolong Tea Reduce Fat Decoction):

Wu Long Cha (Folium Praeparatum Camelliae Sinensis), 15g
He Shou Wu (Radix Polygoni Multiflori), 12g
Dang Shen (Radix Codonopsis), 9g
Bai Zhu (Rhizoma Atractylodis Macrocephalae), 9g
He Ye (Folium Nelumbinis), 9g
Mai Ya (Fructus Germinatus Hordei), 9g
Shan Zha (Fructus Crataegi), 9g
Tu Bei Chong (Eupolyphaga/Steleophaga), 9g

Formula explanation: Within this formula, *Dang Shen* and *Bai Zhu* fortify the spleen and supplement the qi. *Bai Zhu* additionally dries dampness. *Wu Long Cha* powerfully upbears the clear, thus rectifying the qi. It also seeps dampness. It also reduces blood pressure when there is hypertension. *He Ye* clears stomach heat and eliminates dampness. *Mai Ya* disperses food and abducts stagnation and rectifies the qi. *Shan Zha* likewise disperses food and abducts stagnation. However, it also quickens the blood and transforms stasis. *Tu Bei Chong* quickens the blood and transforms stasis, while *He Shou Wu* nourishes the blood. This ingredient helps supplement the qi by nourishing the blood, remembering that the blood is the mother of the qi. This ingredient also helps prevent damage to the righteous from the various attacking and draining medicinals in this formula, especially *Wu Long Cha*. Therefore, this ingredient can also be seen as a harmonizing ingredient in this formula. *Wu Long Cha, Bai Zhu, He Ye, Mai Ya, He Shou Wu,* and *Shan Zha* are all demonstrated antiadiposity ingredients in contemporary Chinese medicine.

For spleen yang vacuity, use *Li Zhong Wan* (Rectify the Center Pills):

Ren Shen (Radix Ginseng), 9-15g
Bai Zhu (Rhizoma Atractylodis Macrocephalae), 9g
Gan Jiang (dry Rhizoma Zingiberis), 6-9g
mix-fried *Gan Cao* (Radix Glycyrrhizae), 3-6g

Formula explanation: *Ren Shen, Bai Zhu,* and mix-fried *Gan Cao* fortify the spleen and supplement the qi. *Gan Jiang* warms yang.

Additions & subtractions: For shortness of breath, fatigue, and spontaneous sweating, add *Huang Qi* (Radix Astragali), 15g. For dampness, add *Fu Ling* (Poria), 12g, and *Ze Xie* (Rhizoma Alismatis), 9g. For profuse phlegm, add

Ban Xia (Rhizoma Pinelliae) and *Chen Pi* (Pericarpium Citri Reticulatae), 9g each. For marked cold with chilled extremities, add *Gui Zhi* (Ramulus Cinnamomi), 9-15g, and *Zhi Fu Zi* (Radix Lateralis Praeparata Aconiti), 3-6g.

Ready-made Chinese medicines: *Liu Jun Zi Wan* (Six Gentlemen Pills) fortify the spleen and supplement the qi as well as transform phlegm and eliminate dampness. For spleen qi vacuity, dampness, and middle burner qi stagnation, use *Xiang Sha Liu Jun Zi Wan* (Auklandia & Amomum Six Gentlemen Pills). For spleen yang vacuity, use *Li Zhong Wan* (Rectify the Center Pills). *Fang Ji Huang Qi Wan* (Stephania & Astragalus Pills) are also available in ready-made form, as are *Wu Long Pian* (Black Dragon Tablets).

Diet & lifestyle: Eat warming, cooked foods and avoid raw and chilled foods. Also avoid too much sugar and sweets as well as too many refined carbohydrates, especially in the form or bread and pasta. According to Chinese medicine, in excess, the sweet flavor damages the spleen and engenders too many fluids. Breads and pastas are called "sodden wheat foods" in Chinese medicine and are also believed to damage the spleen and engender dampness. Use some warming spices, such as black and white pepper, cayenne, cardamom, ginger, and cinnamon. Eat more warm soups and stews.

Get enough exercise to be energized afterwards, not more fatigued. Too much sitting and lying down damage the spleen. Whereas moderate exercise fortifies the spleen and frees the flow of the qi mechanism. Many patients who live a sedentary lifestyle feel too fatigued to exercise. In that case, encourage these patients to take small steps in exercising to build up their qi. Soon they should be able to exercise regularly and will feel more energy overall.

Try not to think too much or worry. According to Chinese medicine, overthinking and worry also damage the spleen. Many patients (overweight or not) worry and obsess about their weight or health and feel overwhelmed by societal and self-induced pressure to lose weight. Some constantly think about calorie-counting. When this kind of thinking and worrying themselves become pathological, they directly work against losing weight.

In patients with spleen qi vacuity, I find regulating the air qi (*kong qi*), a.k.a. the great qi (*da qi*, 大气) through breathing can be extremely helpful in treatment. This is because the spleen and lung qi are mutually interconnected. In Chinese, this kind of practice is called qigong (*qi gong* 气功). For simple instructions on how to do this kind of qigong, see the following table.

1. Lie on your back.
2. Position one hand on the lower abdomen just below the navel.
3. Inhale and exhale a few times. (While the patient breathes, observe the depth of breath into the body. Many people only breathe shallowly into the upper chest. If the patient breathes shallowly, take notice of that and share it with the patient.)
4. Now breathe deeply by inhaling the breath through the nose deep into the abdomen. You should feel the hand on your abdomen rise as the belly expands with the breath. Exhale through the mouth. (Encourage the patient to take a slow, even breath in through the nose. If nasal passages are obstructed, breathing through the mouth is okay.)
5. Inhale through the nose again and, this time, feel the air expand the lungs. Bring the breath through the rib cage then into the abdomen. When the breath fills the abdomen you will again feel your hand rise with it. Exhale through the mouth.
6. Continue inhaling and exhaling in this slow and regulated manner. (Once the patient inhales and exhales a few times, encourage her or him to think about expanding the ribs out to the side with breath as well as pulling the breath deep into the abdomen.)

Ask your patient to talk about how this way of breathing felt different than their uninstructed breathing. Then suggest the practice of this method for at least five minutes per day but advise that 15 minutes is better. I often suggest that my patients try this breathing exercise for the duration of the acupuncture treatment after I insert needles. Most patients become so relaxed after 5-10 minutes that they "forget to breathe" during the rest of the treatment. Their forgetfulness is alright with me because it indicates that the breathing exercise worked well enough for them to relax!

5. Spleen vacuity & stomach heat (*pi xu wei re*, 脾虚胃热)

Signs & symptoms: Obesity, rapid hungering after meals, fatigue, lack of strength, a tendency towards alternating constipation and loose stools, a red facial complexion, a dry mouth with a desire to drink, possibly a bitter taste in the mouth, bad breath, a fat, enlarged tongue with yellow fur, and a slippery, bowstring pulse

Treatment principles: Fortify the spleen and clear the stomach, disperse food and free the flow of the intestines

Acupuncture-moxibustion:
Nei Ting (St 44)
Jie Xi (St 41)
Shang Ju Xu (St 37)
Tai Bai (Sp 3)
Zhong Wan (CV 12)
Tian Shu (St 25)
Da Heng (Sp 15)
Da Chang Shu (Bl 25)

Formula explanation: *Nei Ting, Jie Xie,* and *Shang Ju Xu* clear heat from the stomach and intestines. *Tai Bai* fortifies the spleen and supplements the qi. *Zhong Wan, Tian Shu, Da Heng,* and *Da Chang Shu* clear heat from the stomach and intestines and free the flow of the stools.

Additions & subtractions: For thirst, add *Wei Shu* (Bl 21) and *Fu Liu* (Ki 7). For a bitter taste in the mouth and bad breath, add *Da Ling* (Per 7). For spontaneous hot sweating, add *He Gu* (LI 4).

Chinese herbal formula: Modified *Fei Pang Fang* (Obesity Formula)

Ingredients:
Huang Qi (Radix Astragali), 15g
Ze Xie (Rhizoma Alismatis), 12g
Shan Zha (Fructus Crataegi), 9g
He Ye (Folium Nelumbinis), 9g
Bai Zhu (Rhizoma Atractylodis Macrocephalae), 6g
Fan Xie Ye (Folium Sennae), 3-9g

Formula explanation: *Huang Qi* and *Bai Zhu* fortify the spleen and supplement the qi. *He Ye* clears heat from the stomach. *Shan Zha* abducts stagnation and disperses food, while *Fan Xie Ye* clears heat from the large intestines and frees the flow of the stools. *Ze Xie* seeps dampness, leads yang downward into the yin tract, and leads fluids downward to moisten the intestines.

Additions & subtractions: For severe stomach heat, add *Shi Gao* (Gypsum Fibrosum), 18g, *Zhi Zi* (Fructus Gardeniae), 9g, and *Gan Cao* (Radix Glycyrrhizae), 6g. For severe constipation, add uncooked *Da Huang* (Radix Et Rhizoma Rhei), 6-9g. For damp accumulation with edema in the lower limbs, add *Han Fang Ji* (Radix Stephaniae Tetrandrae), 12g, and *Huang Qi* (Radix Astragali), 15g.

For stomach heat, spleen vacuity, and food stagnation, replace *Fei Pang Fang* with *Xiao Cheng Qi Tang* (Minor Order the Qi Decoction) plus *Bao He Wan* (Preserve Harmony Pills):

Shan Zha (Fructus Crataegi), 9g
Fu Ling (Poria), 9g
Lai Fu Zi (Semen Raphani), 9g
Lian Qiao (Fructus Forsythiae), 9g
Ban Xia (Rhizoma Pinelliae), 9g
uncooked *Da Huang* (Radix Et Rhizoma Rhei), 6-9g
Shen Qu (Massa Medica Fermentata), 6g
Chen Pi (Pericarpium Citri Reticulatae), 6g
Zhi Shi (Fructus Immaturus Aurantii), 6g
Hou Po (Cortex Magnoliae), 6g

Formula explanation: In this case, spleen qi vacuity is minor, while heat and food stagnation are more prominent. *Fu Ling* fortifies the spleen and seeps dampness. *Ban Xia, Hou Po, Zhi Shi,* and *Chen Pi* transform phlegm, eliminate dampness, and downbear turbidity. *Shan Zha, Shen Qu,* and *Lai Fu Zi* abduct stagnation and disperse food. *Lian Qiao* and *Da Huang* clear heat from the stomach and intestines. *Da Huang, Zhi Shi,* and *Hou Po* free the flow of the stools and relieve constipation.

Diet & lifestyle: Follow the instructions for spleen qi vacuity and stomach heat above.

6. Spleen-kidney yang vacuity (*pi shen yang xu,* 脾肾阳虚)

Signs & symptoms: Obesity which is typically more severe below the waist, poor appetite (as long as there is no stomach heat), abdominal distention after eating, fatigued spirit, weakness of the limbs, disliking movement, fear of cold, cold limbs and especially cold feet, short voidings of clear urine or frequent urination, nocturia, decreased libido, low back pain, possible edema in the lower limbs with inhibited urination, loose stools, a pale, enlarged tongue with thin, white fur, and a deep, fine, weak, pulse

Treatment principles: Supplement the kidneys and invigorate yang, fortify the spleen and disperse swelling

Acupuncture-moxibustion:
Guan Yuan (CV 4)
Ming Men (GV 4)

Pi Shu (Bl 20)
Shen Shu (Bl 23)
Zu San Li (St 36)
San Yin Jiao (Sp 6)

Formula explanation: *Zu San Li, Pi Shu,* and *San Yin Jiao* fortify the spleen and supplement the qi. *Guan Yuan, Ming Men, San Yin Jiao,* and *Shen Shu* supplement the kidneys and invigorate yang.

Additions & subtractions: For marked phlegm dampness, add *Feng Long* (St 40) and *Zhong Wan* (CV 12). For concomitant food stagnation, add *Zhong Wan* and *Liang Men* (St 21). For marked water swelling, add *Yin Ling Quan* (Sp 9) and *Shui Fen* (CV 7).

Chinese herbal formula: Modified *Shen Qi Wan* (Kidney Qi Pills)

Ingredients:
Shu Di (cooked Radix Rehmanniae), 18g
Huang Qi (Radix Astragali), 15g
Ze Xie (Rhizoma Alismatis), 12g
Fu Ling (Poria), 12g
Shan Yao (Radix Dioscoreae), 9g
Shan Zhu Yu (Fructus Corni), 9g
Bai Zhu (Rhizoma Atractylodis Macrocephalae), 9g
Gui Zhi (Ramulus Cinnamomi), 9g
Dan Pi (Cortex Moutan), 6g
Zhi Fu Zi (Radix Lateralis Praeparata Aconiti), 6g

Formula explanation: *Huang Qi, Shan Yao, Bai Zhu,* and *Fu Ling* fortify the spleen and supplement the qi. *Shu Di, Shan Zhu Yu,* and *Shan Yao* supplement the kidneys. *Fu Ling* and *Ze Xie* seep dampness, while *Dan Pi* quickens and cools the blood. *Gui Zhi* and *Zhi Fu Zi* warm yang.

Additions & subtractions: For reduced appetite due to concomitant food stagnation, add *Shan Zha* (Fructus Crataegi), 9g. For edema in the lower limbs, add *Han Fang Ji* (Radix Stephaniae Tetrandrae), 9g. For nausea or abdominal distention after meals, add *He Ye* (Folium Nelumbinis), 9g. For liver depression, add *Ju Luo* (Fasciculus Vascularis Citri Reticulatae), 9g, and *Qing Pi* (Pericarpium Citri Reticulatae Viride), 6g.

Ready-made Chinese medicines: *Shen Qi Wan* (Kidney Qi Pills) plus *Si Jun*

Zi Wan (Four Gentlemen Pills) or *Shen Qi Da Bu Wan* (Ginseng & Astragalus Greatly Supplementing Pills)

Diet & lifestyle: Generally follow the instructions for spleen qi vacuity above. While Chinese medicine does describe a number of foods that specifically supplement the kidneys, these are often fatty, high cholesterol foods, such as ham, liver, scallops, and shrimp[12], which are not going to help one lose weight unless eaten very moderately. In general, it is spleen vacuity that eventually leads to kidney vacuity with age, and many Chinese doctors believe that eating a spleen-supplementing diet is the best and safest way to supplement the kidneys via food.

7. Liver depression qi stagnation (*gan yu qi zhi*, 肝郁气滞)

Signs & symptoms: Chest, breast and/or rib-side distention and pain, irritability, burping and hiccup, menstrual irregularities in females, a normal or somewhat dark tongue, and a bowstring pulse. These signs and symptoms tend to manifest or get worse when the patient is under stress or emotionally upset.

Note: This is mainly a textbook pattern in that liver depression rarely presents alone. However, it is one of the most common complicating patterns in all patients who are overweight.

Treatment principles: Course the liver and rectify the qi

Acupuncture-moxibustion:
Tai Chong (Liv 13)
He Gu (LI 4)

Formula explanation: *Tai Chong* and *He Gu* are the four gates which course the liver and rectify the qi, disinhibit the qi mechanism and free the flow of the qi throughout the entire body.

Additions & subtractions: If there is chest oppression add *Dan Zhong* (CV 17) and *Nei Guan* (Per 6). For hiccup or burping, add *Tian Yu* (CV 22) and/or *Zhong Wan* (CV 12) and *Nei Guan*. For breast distention and pain, add *Ru Gen* (St 18), *Dan Zhong, Nei Guan,* and *Zu San Li* (St 36). For rib-side distention and pain, add *Qi Men* (Liv 14) and *Jing Men* (GB 25).

---

12 Shrimp is actually low in total fat and saturated fats. Although it raises LDL by 7% (serving size is 12 large shrimp or 3.5 oz), it raises HDL by 13%. Regular shrimp eaters have reduced triglycerides by 13%. Also it is a great source of Omega-3's, providing 14.8% of D.U. Studies by AHA & published in the *American Journal of Clinical Nutrition* dispell the shrimp/cholesterol/fat myth.

Chinese herbal formula: Modified *Chai Hu Shu Gan San* (Bupleurum Course the Liver Powder)

Ingredients:
Chai Hu (Radix Bupleuri), 9g
Xiang Fu (Rhizoma Cyperi), 9g
Bai Shao (Radix Alba Paeoniae), 9g
Jue Ming Zi (Semen Cassiae), 9g
Zhi Shi (Fructus Immaturus Aurantii), 6g

Formula explanation: *Chai Hu, Xiang Fu,* and *Zhi Shi* course the liver and rectify the qi. *Zhi Shi* also transforms phlegm. *Jue Ming Zi* clears heat from the liver. However, when combined with the above ingredients, it promotes the coursing of the liver and rectification of the qi as well as empirically is known to lower blood pressure and reduce blood lipids. *Bai Shao* nourishes the blood and emolliates the liver. When blood supplements are combined with qi-rectifiers, the ability to resolve depression is improved.

Additions & subtractions: For phlegm qi depression and binding, use *Wen Dan Tang* (Warm the Gallbladder Decoction) instead. This consists of:

Fu Ling (Poria), 12g
Ban Xia (Rhizoma Pinelliae), 9g
Zhu Ru (Caulis Bambusae In Taeniam), 9g
Zhi Ke (Fructus Aurantii), 6-9g
Chen Pi (Pericarpium Citri Reticulatae), 6-9g

Formula explanation: *Fu Ling, Ban Xia, Zhi Ke,* and *Chen Pi* transform phlegm and eliminate dampness. *Ban Xia, Zhi Ke,* and *Chen Pi* also disihibit and free the flow of the qi mechanism and downbear turbidity. *Zhu Ru* courses and clears the liver, transforms phlegm and harmonizes the stomach.

Additions & subtractions: For more marked heat, add *Huang Lian* (Rhizoma Coptidis), 3-6g. For marked dampness and turbidity, add *Shi Chang Pu* (Rhizoma Acori Tatartinowii) and *Huo Xiang* (Herba Pogostemmi), 9g each. For liver-gallbladder damp heat, add *Yin Chen Hao* (Herba Artemisiae Scopariae) and *Huang Qin* (Radix Scutellariae), 9g each.

For phlegm heat harassing the heart resulting in insomnia and heart palpitations, consider *Zhu Ru Wen Dan Tang* (Caulis Bambusae Warm the Gallbladder Decoction):

Chai Hu (Radix Bupleuri), 12g
Xiang Fu (Rhizoma Cyperi), 9g
Zhu Ru (Caulis Bambusae in Taeniam), 9g
Ban Xia (Rhizoma Pinelliae), 9g
Jie Geng (Radix Platycodi), 9g
Fu Ling (Poria), 9g
Ren Shen (Radix Ginseng), 6g
Huang Lian (Rhizoma Coptidis), 6g
Chen Pi (Pericarpium Citri Reticulatae), 6g
Zhi Shi (Fructus Immaturus Citri), 3-6g
Sheng Jiang (uncooked Rhizoma Zingiberis), 2-3 slices
Gan Cao (Radix Glycyrrhizae), 1-3g

Formula explanation: *Chai Hu, Xiang Fu, Zhu Ru, Zhi Shi,* and *Chen Pi* course the liver and resolve depression, the source of depressive heat in most cases of phlegm heat. *Huang Lian* clears heat from the liver-gallbladder, stomach, and heart. *Zhu Ru, Ban Xia, Jie Geng, Fu Ling, Chen Pi, Zhi Shi,* and *Sheng Jiang* transform phlegm and eliminate dampness. In addition, *Jie Geng* guides the other medicinals to the top half of the body and the chest. *Ren Shen* and *Fu Ling* fortify the spleen, supplement the qi, and quiet the spirit. *Gan Cao* harmonizes and regulates all the other medicinals in this formula.

For liver depression, spleen vacuity, stomach heat, and phlegm, use *Xiao Chai Hu Tang* (Minor Bupleurum Decoction):

Chai Hu (Radix Bupleuri), 9g
Dang Shen (Radix Codonopsis), 9g
Ban Xia (Rhizoma Pinelliae), 9g
Huang Qin (Radix Scutellariae), 9g
Sheng Jiang (uncooked Rhizoma Zingiberis), 3 slices
Da Zao (Fructus Jujubae), 3 pieces
mix-fried *Gan Cao* (Radix Glycyrrhizae), 3g

Formula explanation: *Chai Hu* courses the liver and rectifies the qi. *Dang Shen, Da Zao,* and mix-fried *Gan Cao* fortify the spleen and supplement the qi. *Ban Xia* and *Sheng Jiang* transform phlegm, eliminate dampness, and harmonize the stomach. *Huang Qin* clears the stomach.

Additions & subtractions: For more marked spleen qi vacuity, add *Huang Qi* (Radix Astragali), 9-15g, and *Bai Zhu* (Rhizoma Atractylodis Macrocephalae), 9g. For more marked phlegm, add *Ban Xia* (Rhizoma Pinelliae) and *Chen Pi* (Pericarpium Citri Reticulatae), 9g each. For food stagnation, add *Shan Zha* (Fructus Crataegi) and *Lai Fu Zi* (Semen Raphani), 9g each. For more marked heat, add *Huang Lian* (Rhizoma Coptidis), 3-6g. For marked dampness with water swelling, add *Bai Zhu*, 9g, *Fu Ling* (Poria), 9g, *Zhu Ling* (Polyporus), 9g, *Ze Xie* (Rhizoma Alismatis), 9g, and *Gui Zhi* (Ramulus Cinnamomi), 6-9g. For spleen yang vacuity, add *Gan Jiang* (dry Rhizoma Zingiberis) and subtract *Sheng Jiang*. For more marked qi stagnation, add *Xiang Fu* (Rhizoma Cyperi), 9g.

Ready-made Chinese medicines: *Chai Hu Shu Gan Wan* (Bupleurum Course the Liver Pills) plus *Er Chen Wan* (Two Aged [Ingredients] Pills). If there is concomitant food stagnation, also add *Bao He Wan* (Protect Harmony Pills). *Wen Dan Tang Wan* (Warm the Gallbladder Tea Pills) and *Xiao Chai Hu Tang Wan* (Minor Bupleurum Tea Pills) are also available.

Diet & lifestyle: One of the main causes of liver depression is unfulfilled desires. This includes the desire to be thin. Thus such a desire to be thin when one has a constitutional predisposition to be more generously endowed than a runway model can itself work against losing weight. Therefore, one should try to cultivate realistic and obtainable desires, remembering that nothing feeds success like success itself. Further, stress is nothing other than one or many unfulfilled desires, the desire to do or have more than our energy, time, skills, or wealth allow. For general stress reduction, nothing beats a combination of regular exercise and daily deep relaxation. Exercise forcibly moves the qi, while deep relaxation causes the qi to flow freely and easily. If one finds oneself always getting angry, which also damages the liver and leads to depression, then one might consider some short-term therapy or anger management classes.

> When we feel stressed we usually need to reign in our desires for sugar and other "comfort foods."

As for diet, there is not much that we can eat that will directly course the liver and resolve depression. It is said that the sweet flavor relaxes the liver. The problem is that we already tend to overeat sugars and sweets in modern society. Therefore, when we feel stressed we usually need to reign in our desires for sugar and other "comfort foods." If liver depression has transformed heat, then we need to be careful not to eat too many spicy, hot, peppery foods, fried, fatty, greasy foods, or drink too much alcohol. All these things can course the liver and resolve depression in the short-term but can aggravate any evil heat, while fatty foods and alcohol can directly engender dampness and phlegm. Because food stagnation can cause or aggravate liver depression, it is also important not to overeat or eat too many hard-to-digest foods. Based on the dictum, "If the liver is diseased, first treat the spleen," eating a spleen-supplementing diet will indirectly but nevertheless greatly help the liver depression.

8. Blood stasis (*xue yu*, 血瘀)

Signs & symptoms: Obesity, chest and rib-side bitterness and fullness, stomach duct glomus and fullness, static macules on the face region, insomnia, profuse dreams, menstrual irregularities or amenorrhea in females, a dark red tongue with white, possibly thin, slimy fur, and a fine, bowstring pulse

Note: This pattern typically complicates other patterns associated with overweight.

Treatment principles: Quicken the blood and transform stasis, move the qi and transform phlegm

Acupuncture-moxibustion:
Tai Chong (Liv 3)
He Gu (LI 4)
San Yin Jiao (Sp 6)
Xue Hai (Sp 10)
Feng Long (St 40)
Zhong Wan (CV 12)

Formula explanation: *Tai Chong* and *He Gu* are the four bars which course the liver and free the flow of the qi of the entire body. Their inclusion is based on the fact that, "The qi moves the blood." *He Gu, San Yin Jiao,* and *Xue Hai* quicken the blood and transform stasis. *Feng Long* and *Zhong Wan* transform phlegm and eliminate dampness.

Additions & subtractions: If there is food stagnation, add *Liang Men* (St 21) or *Shang Wan* (CV 10) and *Xia Wan* (CV 13). If there is spleen qi vacuity, add *Zu San Li* (St 36). If there is water swelling, add *Yin Ling Quan* (Sp 9). If there is stomach heat, add *Nei Ting* (St 44) and/or *Jie Xie* (St 41). If there is damp heat in the liver-gallbladder, add *Yang Ling Quan* (GB 34).

Chinese herbal formula: Modified *Xiao Yao San* (Rambling Powder)

Ingredients:
Chai Hu (Radix Bupleuri), 9g
Xiang Fu (Rhizoma Cyperi), 9g
Bai Zhu (Rhizoma Atractylodis Macrocephalae), 9g

Fu Ling (Poria), 9g
Ban Xia (Rhizoma Pinelliae), 9g
Hong Hua (Flos Carthami), 9g
Tao Ren (Semen Persicae), 9g
Dang Gui (Radix Angelicae Sinensis), 9g
Chi Shao (Radix Rubra Paeoniae), 9g
Shan Zha (Fructus Crataegi), 6-9g
Jue Ming Zi (Semen Cassiae), 6-9g

Formula explanation: Within this formula, *Chai Hu* and *Xiang Fu* course the liver and rectify the qi. *Hong Hua, Tao Ren, Dang Gui, Chi Shao,* and *Shan Zha* quicken the blood and transform stasis. *Shan Zha* also abducts stagnation and disperses food. *Bai Zhu, Fu Ling,* and *Ban Xia* transform phlegm and eliminate dampness. *Jue Ming Zi* clears the liver if depression has transformed heat and is empirically used to lower blood pressure, reduce blood lipids, and lose weight.

Ready-made Chinese medicines: Consider *Tao Hong Si Wu Tang Wan* (Persica & Carthamus Four Materials Tea Pills) combined with *Er Chen Wan* (Two Aged [Ingredients] Pills) and/or *Xiao Yao Wan* (Rambling Pills).

Diet & lifestyle: Because the qi moves the blood as well as water fluids, exercise is generally good for blood stasis. If the qi moves, the blood moves. Whereas too much sitting and lying about can lead to blood stasis. Other things that can improve the movement of blood are radiant heat saunas, daily self-massage (called *dao yin* in Chinese medicine), professionally administered massage, abdominal massage, and dry-brushing.

9. Damp heat internally brewing (*shi re nei yun*, 湿热内蕴)

Signs & symptoms: Right-sided rib-side distention and pain, ductal and abdominal distention and fullness, palpable pain in the gallbladder area, torpid intake, nausea, vomiting, dry mouth with a bitter taste, thirst with no desire to drink, alternating hot and cold, possible jaundice, dry stools, yellow urine, slimy, yellow tongue fur, and a bowstring, slippery, rapid pulse

Note: This pattern describes acute cholecystitis and cholelithiasis. It is included here because cholecystitis is most commonly seen in the overweight and also to provide space for formulas for chronic cholecystitis associated with being overweight.

Treatment principles: Clear heat and disinhibit dampness, disinhibit the gallbladder and expel stones, free the flow of the interior and attack and precipitate

Acupuncture-moxibustion:
Ri Yue (GB 24), right side
Yang Ling Quan (GB 34)
Zhi Gou (TB 6)
Dan Shu (Bl 19)
Dan Nang Xue (M-LE-23), right side, if tender to palpation

Formula explanation: *Ri Yu* frees the flow of the qi and blood in the channels and network vessels in the rib-side area and stops pain. *Yang Ling Quan, Zhi Gou, Dan Shu*, and *Dan Nang Xue* clear heat and eliminate dampness from the liver-gallbladder, move the qi and stop pain in the rib-side area. *Zhi Gou* and *Yang Ling Quan* also free the flow of the stools.

Additions & subtractions: For severe pain, add *He Gu* (LI 4) and *Qi Men* (Liv 14). For jaundice, add *Zhi Yang* (GV 9). For abdominal distention and pain, add *Zu San Li* (St 36). For nausea and vomiting, add *Nei Guan* (Per 6) and *Zhong Wan* (CV 12). For fever and chills, add *Qu Chi* (LI 11) and *He Gu*.

Chinese herbal formula: Modified *Yin Chen Hao Tang* (Artemesia Scoparia Decoction)

Ingredients:
Yin Chen Hao (Herba Artemesiae Scopariae), 12g
Zhi Zi (Fructus Gardeniae), 9g
uncooked *Da Huang* (Radix Et Rhizoma Rhei), 3-9g

Formula explanation: Within this formula, *Yin Chen Hao* and *Zhi Zi* clear heat and eliminate dampness from the liver-gallbladder. *Yin Chen Hao* also courses the liver and rectifies the qi, thus resolving depression and stopping pain. *Da Huang* clears heat and drains fire by freeing the flow of the stools.

Additions & subtractions: If there is alternating fever and chills, headache, and a bitter taste in the mouth, add *Chai Hu* (Radix Bupleuri) and *Huang Qin* (Radix Scutellariae), 9g each. If there is rib-side pain and abdominal fullness, add *Yu Jin* (Rhizoma Curcumae) and *Zhi Shi* (Fructus Immaturus Aurantii), 9g each. If there is nausea and vomiting, add *Zhu Ru* (Caulis Bambusae In Taeniam) and *Shen Qu* (Massa Medica Fermentata), 9g each. Without constipation, delete *Da Huang*. To expel stones, add *Hai Jin Sha* (Spora Lygodii), 15g, and *Ji Nei Jin* (Endothelium Corneum Gigeriae Galli), 9g. If heat is greater than dampness, add *Lian Qiao* (Fructus Forsythiae), 15g, and *Long Dan Cao* (Radix Genitianae), 9g. If dampness is greater than heat, add *Yi Yi Ren* (Semen Coicis) and *Hua Shi* (Talcum), 15g each, *Ban Xia* (Rhizoma Pinelliae) and *Xing Ren* (Semen Armeniacae), 9g each, and *Hou Po* (Cortex Magnoliae), *Bai Dou Kou* (Fructus Cardamomi), and *Dan Zhu Ye* (Herba Lophatheri), 6g each. If there is jaundice, add *Jin Qian Cao* (Herba Lysimachiae/Desmodii), 25g. If stones obstruct the bile duct, add *Wei Ling Xian* (Radix Clematidis) and *Jin Qian Cao*, 30g each.

For liver-spleen damp heat with blood stasis, use instead *Si Jun Zi Tang* (Four Gentlemen Decoction) plus *Ge Xia Zhu Yu Tang* (Below the Diaphragm Dispel Stasis Decoction) with modifications:

Ban Zhi Lian (Herba Scutellariae Barbatae), 15g
Dang Shen (Radix Codonopsis), 15g
Fu Ling (Poria), 15g
Bai Zhu (Rhizoma Atractylodis Macrocephalae), 9g
Tao Ren (Semen Persicae), 9g
Dang Gui (Radix Angelicae Sinensis), 9g
Yin Chen Hao (Herba Artemesiae Scopariae), 9g
Xiang Fu (Rhizoma Cyperi), 9g
Yan Hu Suo (Rhizoma Corydalis), 9g
Hong Hua (Flos Carthami), 6g
Dan Pi (Cortex Moutan), 6g
Gan Cao (Radix Glycyrrhizae), 3-6g

For dampness and heat damaging qi and yin, use instead *Yi Qi Ruan Gan Tang* (Boost the Qi & Soften the Liver Decoction):

Huang Qi (Radix Astragali), 30g
Sheng Di (uncooked Radix Rehmanniae), 12g
Gou Qi Zi (Fructus Lycii), 12g
Bai Shao (Radix Alba Paeoniae), 12g
Shan Zhu Yu (Fructus Corni), 12g
Yin Chen Hao (Herba Artemesiae Scopariae), 12g
Shan Zha (Fructus Crataegi), 12g
Hu Zhang (Rhizoma Polygoni Cuspidati), 12g
processed *Da Huang* (Radix Et Rhizoma Rhei), 9g
Chen Pi (Pericarpium Citri Reticulatae), 6g
Qing Pi (Pericarpium Citri Reticulatae Viride), 6g
mix-fried *Gan Cao* (Radix Glycyrrhizae), 6g

Ready-made Chinese medicines: *Si Jun Zi Wan* (Four Gentlemen Pills) and

Ge Xia Zhu Yu Wan (Below the Diaphragm Dispel Stasis Pills) are both available for liver-spleen damp heat with blood stasis.

Diet & lifestyle: The foods and drinks which directly internally engender dampness and heat are hot, spicy, peppery foods, fats and oils, including fried foods and dairy products, and alcohol. However, dampness due to overeating sugars and sweets and dampness-engendering foods can combine with depressive heat transformed from liver depression qi stagnation. Therefore, one should also take care with sugars and sweets, fruits and especially fruit juices, and emotional stress and try to get regular physical exercise.

10. Yin vacuity with internal heat (*yin xu nei re*, 阴虚内热)

Signs & symptoms: Obesity, clouded head, blurred vision, head distention, headache, low back pain, aching, and limpness, vexatious heat in the five hearts, a red facial complexion, irritability, vexation and agitation, a red tongue tip with thin fur, and a fine, rapid, slightly bowstring pulse

Note: It is not uncommon to find overweight patients with marked signs and symptoms of yin vacuity. In this case, vacuity and repletion exist at the same time.

Treatment principles: Enrich yin and clear heat at the same time as transforming phlegm

Acupuncture-moxibustion:
Zhong Wan (CV 12)
Feng Long (St 40)
Zu San Li (St 36)
San Yin Jiao (Sp 6)
Tai Xi (Ki 3)

Formula explanation: *Zhong Wan, Zu San Li,* and *Feng Long* transform phlegm and eliminate dampness. *Zu San Li* and *San Yin Jiao* supplement the latter heaven to bolster the former heaven and, thereby, indirectly enrich yin. *San Yin Jiao* and *Tai Xi* supplement the kidneys and directly enrich yin.

Additions & subtractions: For head distention and pain, add *Feng Chi* (GB 21) and *Tai Yang* (M-HN-9). For low back aching and pain, add *Shen Shu* (Bl 23) and *Da Chang Shu* (Bl 25). For irritability, add *Xing Jian* (Liv 2) and *Nei Guan* (Per 6). For heat in the liver, add *Xing Jian* and *Yang Ling Quan* (GB 34). For heat in the stomach, add *Nei Ting* (St 44) and *He Gu* (LI 4). For heat in the large intestine, add *Tian Shu* (St 25) and *Da Chang Shu* (Bl 25).

Chinese herbal formula: Unnamed empirical formula

Ingredients:
Jiao Gu Lan (Herba Gynostemmae Pentaphyllae), 15g
Kun Bu (Thallus Algae), 15g
Hai Zao (Sargassium), 15g
Sheng Di (uncooked Radix Rehmanniae), 12g
Nu Zhen Zi (Fructus Ligustri Lucidi), 12g
Han Lian Cao (Herba Ecliptae), 12g

Formula explanation: Within this formula, *Kun Bu* and *Hai Zao* soften the hard and transform phlegm. *Sheng Di*, *Nu Zhen Zi*, and *Han Lian Cao* supplement the kidneys and enrich yin. *Jiao Gu Lan* clears heat and empirically reduces blood lipids and body fat.

Additions & subtractions: For low back pain, add *Du Zhong* (Cortex Eucommiae) and *Chuan Niu Xi* (Rhizoma Cyathulae), 9g each, and *Sang Ji Sheng* (Herba Taxilli), 12-15g. For head distention and pain, add *Xia Ku Cao* (Spica Prunellae), 15g, and *Gou Teng* (Ramulus Uncariae Cum Uncis) and *Tian Ma* (Rhizoma Gastrodiae), 9-12g each. To clear heat more, add *Huang Qin* (Radix Scutellariae), 9g. To subdue yang and downbear counterflow, add *Mu Li* (Concha Ostreae) and *Long Gu* (Os Fossilis Mastodi), 12-15g each. If there is constipation, add uncooked *Da Huang* (Radix Et Rhizoma Rhei), 3-6g.

Ready-made Chinese medicines: Consider *Tian Ma Gou Teng Yin Wan* (Gastrodia & Uncaria Tea Pills) plus *Er Chen Wan* (Two Aged [Ingredients] Pills) if there is yin vacuity with ascendant liver yang hyperactivity and phlegm or *Zhi Bai Di Huang Wan* (Anemarrhena & Phellodendron Rehmannia Pills) plus *Er Chen Wan* (Two Aged [Ingredients] Pills) if there is yin vacuity with effulgent heat and phlegm.

Diet & lifestyle: Dealing with yin vacuity internal heat while overweight can provide some special challenges. Typically, the foods one would normally eat for yin vacuity are contraindicated when there is too much phlegm and dampness. This is because these foods tend to strongly engender fluids and dampness which is nothing other than untransformed fluids. Therefore, the safest and best way via diet to deal with yin vacuity in those who are overweight is to follow a spleen-supplementing diet. To treat the internal heat, one should avoid or minimize hot, spicy, peppery foods, fats and oils, and alcohol and eat a modicum of lettuce, celery, melon, and other cooling foods.

One should also avoid tobacco-smoking and coffee and tea drinking to excess. Coffee and tea are acrid, windy "foods" according to Chinese medicine which can easily damage yin. One should also take special care not to use over-the-counter (OTC) or prescription stimulants if one is yin vacuous.

In the case of yin vacuity, it is also important not to be too active. This means not too physically active but especially not too mentally and emotionally active. In Chinese medicine, activity is referred to as stirring (*dong*, 动), and too much stirring consumes and damages yin. The trick here is to get enough physical exercise to move and transform phlegm and dampness, but not too much mental and emotional stimulation to further cause damage and detriment to yin. Daily deep relaxation is an excellent way to calm down an overactive, overheated mind.

Ear acupuncture

As most readers of this book probably know, ear acupuncture (a.k.a. auriculotherapy) has been widely used in China and the West for the promotion of weight loss. Such ear acupuncture can consist of 0.5 inch fine needles inserted in the ear(s) either daily or every other day or press needles which are inserted and then left for several days, with the patient pressing each needle several times throughout each day. In some cases, tiny ear seeds (either made from real plant seeds or small, round metal spheres, so-called ion pellets) may be used instead of press needles. In that case, the seeds or spheres are taped over the ear points and then the patient presses these several times per day.

Ear acupuncture can and has been used alone or in combination with body acupuncture. In the West, where patients typically cannot come every or every other day for treatment, ear acupuncture is often used "to bridge the gap" between regularly scheduled in-office treatments with body acupuncture. In that case, body acupuncture is scheduled once or twice a week and press needles or seeds are used at ear points in order to continue treatment between scheduled appointments.

It is believed that ear acupuncture can reduce one's appetite and cravings as well as improve the function of specific organs and organ systems. From a review of the Chinese ear acupuncture weight loss research, the main points used for weight loss include:

1. Mouth   4. Shen Men
2. Hunger   5. Brain
3. Endocrine   6. Subcortex

These points are meant to suppress appetite and cravings and increase the metabolism. Two to three of these points are usually combined with 2-3 of the following points based on the Chinese medical pattern discrimination:

1. Stomach
2. Spleen
3. Kidneys
4. Liver

5. Large Intestine
6. Triple Burner
7. Lungs

Altogether, typically 5-6 points are used per treatment. Needles may either be divided between the two ears or all needles may be inserted in only one ear. In the first case, whatever points were needled in the right ear are needled in the left the next treatment and vice versa. In the second case, points are alternated from ear to ear from treatment to treatment. Such alternation prevents "point fatigue."

Unfortunately, many Western patients believe that all that is necessary for acupuncture weight loss is a couple press needles inserted in their ear. As previously stated, this is far from the truth.

However, when combined with diet, exercise, and lifestyle modification, ear acupuncture can be a useful and effective therapy.

Treatments & medicinals to be careful with

According to Chinese medicine, preservation of the essence and qi are crucial to good health. Unfortunately, there are a number of OTC herbal weight-loss remedies which may damage and cause detriment to the essence and qi. In general, such potentially dangerous herbal weight-loss products contain primarily three classes of medicinals when analyzed from the Chinese medical point of view:

1. Attacking and precipitating medicinals (*gong xia yao* 攻下药)
2. Dampness-seeping medicinals (*shen shi yao* 渗湿药)
3. Exterior-resolving medicinals (*jie biao yao* 解表药)

Attacking and precipitating medicinals refer to harsh laxatives, such as *Da Huang* (Radix Et Rhizoma Rhei) and *Fan Xie Ye* (Folium Sennae). Over or inappropriate use of such harsh laxatives purge essential nutrients from the body. Of course one will lose weight because one is not getting adequate nutrition. However, long-term, this is a very dangerous and deleterious way of losing weight similar in approach to the purging of bulimia. Dampness-seeping medicinals are diuretics, such as *Ze Xie* (Rhizoma Alismatis), *Che Qian Zi* (Semen Plantaginis), and *Han Fang Ji* (Radix Stephaniae Tetrandrae). Over or inappropriate use of these may cause dehydration, electrolyte imbalance, and renal dysfunction. Again, such an approach alone or long-term is not a good one. Exterior-resolving medicinals are yang-upbearing and out-thrusting diaphoretics. The most commonly used such diaphorectic in OTC weight loss products was *Ma Huang* (Herba Ephedrae) until the FDA banned its use. *Ma Huang* is a stimulant which increases the body's metabolic rate. Unfortunately, when used in excess or inappropriately, *Ma Huang* plunders yin and damages the righteous qi, and readers are, I am sure, aware of the several deaths attributed in the U.S. to *Ma Huang* in OTC weight loss products.

What I am talking about here is OTC weight-loss aids which are made up only of such attacking and draining herbal medicinals and/or when they are administered without a proper Chinese medical pattern discrimination. As the reader will see, representatives of each of these three categories of medicinals (including each of the medicinals mentioned above) are copiously represented in the above formulas in this chapter. In and of themselves, there is nothing wrong with *Ze Xie, Ma Huang,* or *Da Huang.* The issue is to use them in the right amounts, for the right period of time, in patients presenting the right patterns.

Not only can such OTC weight-loss remedies be dangerous, but, in my experience, they are rarely or, at best, marginally effective. Any weight loss achieved is easily gained back when the product is stopped or when the patient resumes their previous unhealthy eating habits and/or gives up exercising. Bottom line, there is no magic bullet or pill for weight loss in spite of how compelling the packaging looks or spokesperson looks or sounds. Rather than pursuing futile efforts with these ineffective or dangerous OTC products and fad diets, I believe practitioners and their patients should proactively design an individually tailored program integrating a variety of balanced, healthy, safe, and effective therapies. That is why practitioners of traditional Chinese medicine always base treatment on each patient's personally presenting pattern(s). In Chinese, this is called *bian zheng lun zhi* (辨证论治). This is what allows us to tailor the treatment to fit the patient and what makes Chinese medicine the safe, effective, holistic medicine it is.

> Not only can such OTC weight-loss remedies be dangerous, but, in my experience, they are rarely or, at best, marginally effective.

Recently Published Research on the Chinese Medical Treatment of Obesity

5

More than 100 clinical trials have been conducted in China on the Chinese medical treatment of obesity over the last 40 years. Some of these clinical trials involved body acupuncture, others involved ear acupuncture, some involved internally administered Chinese herbal medicine, and yet others involved a combination of body and ear acupuncture or acupuncture and internally administered Chinese herbal medicine. I believe these clinical trials are important for two reasons. First, they prove that Chinese medicine is effective for the treatment of obesity, and secondly, they show how obesity is being treated in China today. The following abstracts have been translated by Bob Flaws, Honora Lee Wolfe, and Robert Helmer. Each gives a reproducible account of the treatment methods used. All this research was conducted and published from 2002-2006. These abstracts are just a small fraction of the total research done in China on obesity and weight loss using acupuncture and Chinese herbal medicine.

1. On pages 50-51 of issue #10, 2004 of *Xin Zhong Yi (New Chinese Medicine)*, Tang Qing-fen et al. of the First Affiliated Hospital of the Guangzhou University of Chinese Medicine & Medicinals published an article titled, "An Analysis of the Therapeutic Effects of Treating 50 Cases of Simple Obesity with *Fei San Zhen* (Fat Three Needles)."

Cohort description
All 50 patients enrolled in this study were seen as outpatients at the Chinese authors' hospital in Guangzhou. Among them, there were 18 males and 32 females 16-55 years of age. These patients had suffered from obesity for from

3-20 years. All were physically overweight. They either ate profusely and easily hungered or ate scantily but were still fat. Other accompanying signs and symptoms included duct and abdominal distention and fullness, constipation, encumbered, fatigued extremities, a normal or slightly red tongue body with thin, yellow fur, and a slippery, forceful pulse or a pale tongue with thin, white fur, and a deep, fine pulse. Forty of the patients had previously taken appetite suppressants and 17 had taken weight loss medications, but had been ineffective. Those who were slightly overweight were 20-30% over their ideal body/mass index (BMI). Those who were moderately overweight were 31-50% over their ideal BMI, and those who were severely overweight were more than 50% over their ideal BMI.

Treatment method
Fei San Zhen consisted of:

Zhong Wan (CV 12)
Dai Mai (GB 26)
Zu San Li (St 36)

Acupuncture was performed using 30 gauge Hua Tuo Brand fine needles. *Zhong Wan* and *Zu San Li* were needled perpendicularly to a depth of 1.2 inches using a 1.5 inch needle. After obtaining the qi, twisting draining technique with large amplitude was used to produce a strong needle sensation. *Dai Mai* was needled with a four inch needle. After obtaining the qi, the needles were connected to a 6805-1 electroacupuncture machine with a dense dispersing wave and as strong a stimulation as the patient could bear. These needles were retained for 40 minutes, and one such treatment was administered every other day. Ten treatments equaled one course of therapy, and a successive three courses were given.

Study outcomes
Outcomes criteria were based on the 1991 National Integrated Chinese-Western Medicine Symposium on Obesity. Cure was defined as loss of weight to one's ideal BMI. Marked effect was defined as loss of 5kg or more. Some effect was defined as loss of 3kg or more. No effect meant that any weight loss was less than 3kg. Based on these criteria, 10 cases were judged cured, 19 cases got a marked effect, 15 cases got some effect, and six cases got no effect. Therefore, the total effectiveness rate was published as 88%.

Discussion
According to the Chinese authors, the main cause of this condition is eating too much and insufficient exercise and physical activity. In terms of Chinese

medical theory, the main viscera involved with this condition are the spleen-stomach, liver, and kidneys. This condition is closely associated with loss of normalcy of the spleen and stomach's movement and transformation. In general, it should be treated by regulating and rectifying the spleen and stomach, upbearing the clear and downbearing turbidity. *Fei San Zhen* is a protocol developed at the Guangzhou University of Chinese Medicine & Medicinals. Within it, *Zu San Li* is the uniting point of the foot yang ming stomach channel. It is also the stomach's lower uniting point. Needling it courses and regulates the yang ming channel qi, frees the flow and regulates the stomach and intestines. *Zhong Wan* is categorized as the stomach's mu or so-called alarm point. It is chosen as a local point in the abdominal region. Needling it perpendicularly regulates and rectifies the spleen-stomach's digestive function. *Dai Mai* is located in the center of the low back and abdomen (meaning at the meeting place of the low back and lower abdomen) where, like a belt or cinch, it controls the circulation of qi of the entire body. According to Drs. Tang *et al.*, when the abdomen is too fat, the dai mai is too tight and, therefore, is not able to control the function of descending and downbearing. Using electroacupuncture at this point is able to ease and free the flow of the dai mai channel qi. When patients undergo this therapy at the same time, as eating less and getting more exercise, it achieves a high rate of success.

2. In issue #7, 2002 of *Xin Zhong Yi (New Chinese Medicine)*, Zou Jun published an article titled, "A Survey of the Treatment Efficacy of Acupuncture and Herbs Combined with Pattern Discrimination in the Treatment of 210 Cases of Simple Obesity." This article appeared on pages 49-50 of that journal.

Cohort description

There were 210 patients in this study, all of whom were 20% or more over their ideal BMI. Patients with secondary obesity or who had accompanying heart, liver, or kidney disease were excluded as were pregnant and breast-feeding women. In addition, patients were excluded if they had a recent history of using cholesterol-lowering medications. Among these 210 patients, there were 80 males and 130 females aged 5-63 years, with an average age of 28.53 years. Their course of disease ranged from one half year to 25 years, with an average duration of three years and two months. Sixty cases exhibited a pattern of stomach heat with damp obstruction, 55 cases manifested a pattern of spleen-kidney dual vacuity, 50 cases presented with liver depression qi stagnation, and 45 cases exhibited yin vacuity with internal heat signs and symptoms.

Treatment method

1. Stomach heat & damp obstruction

The symptoms seen in this group included obesity, head distention, dizziness, rapid hungering after eating, heaviness of the limbs which caused them to be indolent, oral thirst, a predilection for drinking, constipation, a red tongue with slimy, slight yellow fur, and a slippery, slightly rapid pulse. The treatment principles were to clear heat and eliminate dampness. The medicinals used consisted of:

Dan Shen (Radix Salviae Miltiorrhizae)
Ze Xie (Rhizoma Alismatis)
Fu Ling (Poria)
Bai Mao Gen (Rhizoma Imperatae)
Da Huang (Radix Et Rhizoma Rhei)
Shan Zha (Fructus Crataegi)

The acupuncture points chosen were:

Tian Shu (St 25)
Shang Ju Xu (St 37)
Gong Sun (Sp 4)

2. Spleen-kidney dual vacuity

This group presented with obesity, fatigue, lack of strength, low back ache, lower leg limpness, impotence, chilled genitalia, a pale red tongue with white fur, and a deep, fine, forceless pulse. The treatment principles were to warm the kidneys and fortify the spleen. The medicinal used consisted of:

Zhi Fu Zi (Radix Lateralis Praeparata Aconiti)
Rou Gui (Cortex Cinnamomi)
Du Zhong (Cortex Eucommiae)
Bai Zhu (Rhizoma Atractylodis Macrocephalae)
Fu Ling (Poria)
He Ye (Folium Nelumbinis)
Jiao Gu Lan (Herba Gynostemmae Pentaphyllae)

The acupuncture points chosen were:

Pi Shu (Bl 20)
Shen Shu (Bl 23)
San Yin Jiao (Sp 6)

3. Liver depression qi stagnation

The signs and symptoms listed for this pattern were obesity, chest and rib-side bitterness and fullness, stomach duct glomus and fullness, static macules on the face region, insomnia, profuse dreams, menstrual irregularities or amenorrhea in females, a dark red tongue with white, possibly thin, slimy fur, and a fine, bowstring pulse, for which the treatment principles were to rectify the qi and quicken the blood. The medicinals used for these purposes included:

Chai Hu (Radix Bupleuri)
Xiang Fu (Rhizoma Cyperi)
Bai Zhu (Rhizoma Atractylodis Macrocephalae)
Hong Hua (Flos Carthami)
Tao Ren (Semen Persicae)
Shan Zha (Fructus Crataegi)
Cao Jue Ming (Semen Cassiae)

The acupuncture points chosen were:

Tai Chong (Liv 3)
San Yin Jiao (Sp 6)
He Gu (LI 4)

4. Yin vacuity with internal heat

This group manifested the signs and symptoms of obesity, clouded head, blurred vision, head distention, headache, low back pain, aching, and limpness, vexatious heat in the five hearts, low-grade fever, a red tongue tip with thin fur, and a fine, rapid, slightly bowstring pulse. The treatment principles were to enrich yin and clear heat, and the medicinals used included:

Kun Bu (Thallus Algae)
Hai Zao (Sargassium)
Jiao Gu Lan (Herba Gynostemma Pentaphyllae)
Sheng Di (uncooked Radix Rehmanniae)
Nu Zhen Zi (Fructus Ligustri Lucidi)
Han Lian Cao (Herba Ecliptae)

The acupuncture points chosen were:

Zhong Wan (CV 12)
Zu San Li (St 36)
Tai Xi (Ki 3)

The above Chinese medicinals were made into gelatin capsules, each of which weighed 0.3 grams. Three of these capsules were administered each time, three times each day. Acupuncture was administered bilaterally once each day. Twenty-one days equaled one course of treatment, and results were assessed after completing two courses. In addition, patients were instructed to press pellets taped over ear points three times per day, but these ear points were not specified in the article.

Study outcomes

Marked effect was defined as a reduction in body weight of 5kg or more or a reduction in BMI of 5% or more. Some effect meant that there was a loss of 3kg of weight or more or a reduction in BMI of 5%. No effect meant that there was less than a 3kg loss in weight or less than a 5% reduction in BMI. Based on these criteria, 81 patients were judged to have gotten a marked effect, 91 got some effect, and 38 got no effect, for a total amelioration rate of 81.9%. In terms of outcomes between the different groups of patterns, these were more or less the same. There were also statistically significant changes ($P \geq 0.01$) in mean total cholesterol, triglycerides, and high density lipoproteins in all groups of patterns from before to after treatment.

Discussion

According to Dr. Zou, obesity is mainly related to diet, constitution, lack of sufficient exercise, and emotional factors. Dr. Zou believes that the root of obesity is vacuity and its tips or branches are repletion. In terms of root vacuities, these are spleen loss of movement and transformation and kidney loss of warming, shining, enriching, and moistening. The branch repletions are phlegm dampness internally obstructing and qi mechanism obstruction and stagnation. Therefore, Dr. Zou divides the treatment of this condition into the four patterns of stomach heat with damp obstruction, spleen-kidney dual vacuity, liver depression qi stagnation, and yin vacuity with internal heat. According to Dr. Zou most Chinese medical weight loss regimes attempt to treat all patients with obesity with a single medicine or treatment method. However, this has not produced consistently high results. Rather, Dr. Zou finds that treating on the basis of individual pattern discrimination is able to achieve better results.

3. In issue #1, 2003 of the *Bei Jing Zhong Yi Za Zhi (Beijing Journal of Chinese Medicine)*, Zhang Lu published an article titled, "Acupuncture on Spleen & Stomach Channel and Ren Mai Channel Points in the Treatment of 40 Cases of Stomach & Intestinal Replete Heat Pattern Simple Obesity." This article appeared on pages 41-42 of that journal.

Cohort description

There were 33 females and seven males among the 40 patients described in this study. The youngest of these patients was 16 and the oldest was 47 years old, with an average age of 32.5 years. The shortest disease duration was two years and the longest was 18 years. All these patients were seen as outpatients at the Acupuncture Department of the Beijing Chinese Medicine Hospital. Diagnostic criteria was based on guidelines issued by the Chinese National People's Ministry of Health & Hygiene in 1995 in *Zhong Yao Xin Yao Zhi Liao Fei Pang Bing De Lin Chuang Zhi Dao Yuan Ze (Clinical References & Principles for the Treatment of Obesity with Chinese Medicinals & New Medications)*, second edition, pages 175-177. This included a body mass index of more than 20% over ideal with a percentage of fat of more than 30%. In terms of the pattern discrimination of replete heat in the stomach and intestines, the main presenting signs and symptoms included bodily obesity, excessive eating and easy hunger, oral thirst with a predilection to drinking, constipation, short, reddish urination, a red tongue with yellow fur, and a bowstring, rapid, slippery pulse.

Treatment method

The main points needled on all 40 patients consisted of:

Tian Shu (St 25)
Zu San Li (St 36)
Nei Ting (St 44)
Feng Long (St 40)
Shang Ju Xu (St 37)
Yin Ling Quan (Sp 9)
San Yin Jiao (Sp 6)
Da Heng (Sp 15)
Shang Wan (CV 13)
Zhong Wan (CV 12)
Xia Wan (CV 10)

If there was mainly lower abdominal obesity, *Fu Jie* (Sp 14) was added bilaterally. If there was mainly obesity of the thighs, *Ji Men* (Sp 11) was added bilaterally. Draining method was used on all points. This consisted of relatively rapid, large amplitude twisting and turning technique to produce a strong subjective needle sensation. In addition, most of the patients also received electro-acupuncture stimulation. Needles were retained for 30 minutes each treatment, and 10 days of treatment equaled one course. Typically, treatment involved six such courses.

Study outcomes

Clinical control meant that the body weight dropped to normal levels or was within normal parameters. Marked effect was defined as a drop in body weight of 5kg or more and a reduction in percentage of fat of 5% or more. Some effect meant that body weight dropped 3kg or more and percentage of fat and any associated clinical symptoms decreased. No effect meant that there was no reduction in either body weight or percentage of fat. Based on these criteria, after 1-4 courses of treatment, two cases (5%) were clinically controlled. These two cases had a percentage of fat reduction of up to 30%. Twenty-five cases (62.5%) were judged to have experienced a marked effect, with 13 cases seeing a 9-10% reduction in percentage of fat and 12 cases a 5-8% reduction in percentage of fat. Ten cases (25%) got some effect. These patients experienced a 2-5% reduction in percentage of fat. Three cases (7.5%) got no result. Therefore, the total effectiveness rate was calculated as 92.5%.

Discussion

According to Dr. Zhang, many cases of simple obesity present a pattern of stomach-intestine replete heat. This is due to replete heat accumulating and stagnating in the intestinal tract. Therefore, treatment should mainly regulate and rectify the spleen and stomach. Such patients are habitually bodily yang exuberant and their digestive function is excessively strong. In this case, regulating and rectifying the spleen and stomach clears heat and downbears turbidity, frees the flow of the bowels and transforms fat. *Zu San Li* is the uniting point of the stomach, while *Shang Ju Xu* is the uniting point of the large intestine. Needling these two points at the same time drains heat from these two channels. Similarly, draining *Nei Ting* also drains stomach channel heat. Based on the saying, "People [who are] fat [have] lots of phlegm [and] dampness," *Yin Ling Quan* is used to drain dampness, while *Feng Long* in combination with *Zhong Wan* is used to transform phlegm. *San Yin Jiao* is chosen to regulate the three yin and thereby balance the metabolism of the entire body. In addition, needling the three ducts (*i.e.*, *Shang Wan*, *Zhong Wan*, and *Xia Wan*) regulates and slows the stomach's peristalsis. Heavy hand technique and strong stimulation is used based on the saying, "All repletions [should be] drained." This needling technique is also based on the saying from the chapter titled, "Normal & Counterflow, Fat & Thin," from the *Ling Shu (Spiritual Axis)*, "[For those whose] age [and bodily] substance are strong and large, [whose] qi and blood are full and exuberant, [whose] skin is drum-like, hard, and secure, [and whose disease] is due to the addition of evils, needling should be deep with retention, such as fat people." At the same time as undergoing the above treatment, patients should be counseled to eat less high heat foods as well as less high fat foods. They should eat more greens, vegetables, and fruits. Likewise, they should lower their intake of salt and get more physical exercise. According to Dr. Zhang, when patients follow this regime, one can definitely improve the effectiveness rate of the above acupuncture protocol.

When the stomach is hot, it means its function is hyperactive. Because every person is different, some people constitutionally have hot stomachs. Stomach heat can also be created by eating foods that are greasy and fatty as well as foods which are acrid and hot in flavor and nature, such as many cooking spices. The stomach's function is to rotten and ripen foods and liquids taken in and to downbear the turbid. The Chinese character for "ripen" (*shu* 熟) is the same character as for "to cook." Therefore, the function of the stomach is likened to the cooking of a pot, fermentation tun, or still. Because a hot stomach burns through foods and liquids more quickly than normal, the appetite is large. However, overeating leads to food stagnation which, in turn, increases the engenderment and transformation of depressive heat. Food stagnation jams the qi mechanism and impairs the spleen's control over the movement and transformation of water fluids. Therefore, the clear and turbid are not completely and correctly separated and phlegm and dampness collect and accumulate. Since the spleen is averse to dampness, this internally engendered dampness damages the spleen. It is interesting that the average age of patients in this study was 32.5 years and that the majority of these patients were female. Females typically become spleen vacuous sometime in their mid 30s and are more prone to spleen vacuity than males due to the demands of menstruation, gestation, and lactation. Depressive heat damages fluids and engenders dryness, thus causing intestinal dryness and constipation. Patients with replete heat in the stomach and intestines also commonly have facial acne along the course of the hand and foot yang ming. Although Dr. Zhang focused his sole attention on the spleen, stomach, and large intestine, in real life, this scenario is commonly complicated by liver depression qi stagnation.

4. On page 39 of issue #1, 2005 of the *Zhen Jiu Lin Chuang Za Zhi (Clinical Journal of Acupuncture & Moxibustion)*, Guo Xiao-yun published an article titled, "Clinical Observations of the Treatment of Simple Obesity with Abdominal Needling & TDP Illumination."

Cohort description

There were two males and 28 females enrolled in this study for a total of 30 patients. All had a body mass index (BMI) of 28.0 or higher. Therefore, all met the criterion for obesity. All were seen as outpatients at the Guangzhou Municipal No. 2 People's Hospital in Guangdong. Patients with secondary obesity were excluded from this study.

Treatment method

The points chosen consisted of:

Zhong Wan (CV 12)
Xia Wan (CV 10)
Qi Hai (CV 6)
Guan Yuan (CV 4)
Hua Rou Men (St 24)
Da Heng (Sp 15)

Hua Tuo Brand 0.25 x 40mm sterile disposable needles were used to needle these points. They were needled perpendicularly to a relatively deep level. Slow twisting and turning hand technique was used to move, hasten, and obtain the qi. Then the needles were passively retained without further movement. During that time, a TDP lamp was used to shine on *Shen Que* (CV 8) with as hot a degree of heat the patient could bear. One such treatment was done per day lasting 30 minutes each time. After five days of treatment, there was a two day rest. Ten such treatments equaled one course of therapy, after which seven days of rest was given. Altogether, three such courses were administered.

Study outcomes

Cure was defined as a reduction of BMI to within normal parameters. Marked effect meant that the patient lost 5kg or more. Some effect meant that the patient lost 3kg or more, and no effect meant that the patient lost less than 3kg. Based on these criteria, four cases were judged cured, 10 got a marked effect, 13 got some effect, and only three got no effect. Therefore, the total effectiveness rate was reported as 90%. Of the three cases who got no effect, two cases lost one pound and 1.4 pounds. The other case was a woman who was six months postpartum. During the course of treatment, this woman ate 250ml of fresh yogurt each night which is why, the author believes, she lost no weight.

Discussion

According to the author, in Chinese medicine, simple obesity is mainly due to yang qi vacuity weakness, loss of regulation of the function of the viscera and bowels, loss of duty of the qi mechanism's upbearing and downbearing, entering and exiting, and uneasy movement of the blood. This then results in phlegm dampness and stasis obstruction with fat and turbidity internally filling the body and flesh. Needling the above points on the abdomen regulates and disciplines the viscera and bowels, channels and network vessels as well as spreads and extends the qi and blood to the entire body of the patient. *Da Heng* dispels dampness and fortifies the spleen. *Zhong Wan* and *Xia Wan* regulate the middle burner, regulate upbearing and downbearing, and also eliminate phlegm and dampness. Together, the author believes these points promote the normal metabolism of fat. *Qi Hai* supplements the qi, while *Guan Yuan* supplements and boosts the yang qi. These points also free the flow and spread the yang qi so as to also metabolize fat. Finally, *Hua Rou Men*, a point on the stomach channel, when combined with the preceding points is wondrous for freeing the flow of the bowels. Stimulating the abdomen with a TDP lamp increases and strengthens the actions of all these points.

5. On page 35 of issue #12, 2004 of *Gan Su Zhong Yi (Gansu Chinese Medicine)*, Sun Li published an article titled, "A Short Discussion of the Acupuncture-moxibustion Treatment of 20 Cases of Simple Obesity."

Cohort description

Of the 20 patients enrolled in this study, only one was a male. The oldest patient was 52 and the youngest was 11 years old. Seven cases were grade I overweight (meaning a BMI equal to or more than 25 but less than 30). Twelve patients were grade II overweight (meaning a BMI equal to or more than 30 and less than 35), and one patient was grade III overweight (meaning a BMI equal to or more than 35 but less than 40). All patients in this study met WHO diagnostic criteria for being overweight. Patients whose obesity was secondary to disease were excluded from this study.

Treatment method

Body acupuncture consisted of the following main points:

Tian Shu (St 25)
Xia Wan (CV 10)
Shi Men (CV 5)
Da Ju (St 27)

Auxiliary points consisted of:

Zu San Li (St 36)
San Yin Jiao (Sp 6)
Feng Long (St 40)
Qu Chi (LI 11)
Nei Guan (Per 6)
He Gu (LI 4)

One and a half inch fine needles were used to needle these points. After obtaining the qi, draining technique was used with strong stimulation. The needles were stimulated every 10 minutes while in place, and they were retained for 30 minutes each treatment. One such treatment was done per day, with 10 treatments equaling one course of therapy. After withdrawing the needles, the abdomen was massaged using several different manipulations for an unspecified period of time.

Ear acupuncture consisted of the following main points:

1. Endocrine   4. Hunger
2. Three Burners 5. Mouth
3. Subcortex   6. Brain

Auxiliary ear points included:

1. Stomach   4. Lungs
2. Liver   5. Large Intestine
3. Kidneys

Depending on the patient's pattern discrimination and condition, *Wang Bu Liu Xing* (Semen Vaccariae) seeds were taped over several of these points which the patient was instructed to press 40-50 times each day, pressing until the ear became red and hot. These points were alternated from one ear to the other once every three days. It was forbidden to use points on both ears at the same time.

Study outcomes

Cure was defined as achievement of a BMI of less than 25 after treatment. Marked effect was defined as a weight loss of more than 5kg. Some effect was defined as a weight loss of 2kg or more, and no effect meant that there was no improvement in weight. Based on these criteria, three cases (15%) were judged cured, 11 cases (55%) got a marked effect, and six cases (30%) got some effect. Thus the total effectiveness rate was 100%.

Discussion

According to Dr. Sun, in Chinese medicine, fat is categorized as a species of "heavy phlegm, turbidity, and dampness." It is formed due to non-transformation of righteous fluids and humors. These collect and accumulate and produce fat. For instance, if the three burners' qi transformation does not diffuse due to the lungs, spleen, and/or kidneys' regulation, movement, conduction, transportation, streaming, and transforming losing their duty, there will be yang vacuity and yin exuberance. Water rheum and phlegm turbidity collect internally, and this leads to the creation of fat. Thus we can see that obesity is closely associated with loss of regulation of the lungs, spleen, kidneys, and three burners, and, of these, it is most closely associated with the spleen. Therefore, within the above protocol, the main points are all located on the foot yang ming stomach channel, the foot tai yin spleen channel, and the conception vessel. These points are able to fortify the spleen and boost the stomach, transform phlegm and eliminate dampness. Massage on the abdominal region can course and free the flow of the spleen-stomach channel and network vessel qi and blood, disperse food and abduct stagnation, and stimulate the metabolism. A large amount of scientific research has made it clear that the combination of body acupuncture and ear acupuncture can increase and strengthen the body's hypophysal-pituitary-adrenal cortex and sympathetic-adrenal system functions, thus promoting the body's metabolism of fat as well as controlling appetite. Therefore, Dr. Sun believes that the combination of body and ear acupuncture for the treatment of simple obesity is quite good. In addition, it is without side effects.

6. On page 19 of issue #1, 2005 of the *Zhen Jiu Lin Chuang Za Zhi (Clinical Journal of Acupuncture & Moxibustion)*, Qu Ben-qi et al. published an article titled, "The Acupuncture, Ear Point Pressure & Dietary Regulation Treatment of 268 Cases of Obesity."

Cohort description

All 268 patients enrolled in this study were seen as outpatients at a university-affiliated hospital in Shandong. Among them, there were 238 females and only 30 males. These patients ranged in age from 16-52 years. Most had already tried weight reduction medications without success.

Treatment method
Body acupuncture consisted of needling the following points:

Qu Chi (LI 11)
Yang Ling Quan (GB 34)
Feng Long (St 40)
Tai Chong (Liv 3)
Shang Ju Xu (St 37)
Zhong Wan (CV 12)
Tian Shu (St 25)
Shui Fen (CV 9)
Liang Men (St 21)
Hua Rou Men (St 24)
Da Heng (Sp 15)

After obtaining the qi, the needles were retained for 30 minutes, They were stimulated every 10 minutes. Depending on the patient's condition, either supplementing or draining hand technique was used. During the first course of treatment, acupuncture was given once per day. During the second and third courses, it was given once every other day. Altogether, 30 treatments were administered.

Ear points chosen consisted of:

1. Mouth   5. Shen Men
2. Lungs   6. Endocrine
3. Stomach   7. Hunger
4. Triple Burner

Magnetic pellets were taped over 4-5 of these points on one ear at a time. Every three days, the ears were switched. Each day, patients were instructed to press these pellets 2-3 times for 5-10 minutes each time.

At the same time, patients were instructed to control their intake of sugar and fats and to eat more vegetables and low-sugar fruits.

Study outcomes
After three courses of treatment, the most a patient lost was 20 pounds and

the least was 2.5 pounds. After the first course of treatment, the most a single patient lost was eight pounds, and the least was two pounds. No other outcomes were provided.

Discussion
According to the Chinese authors of this study, obesity is due to former heaven natural endowment insufficiency, addiction to fatty, sweet, thick, slimy foods, enduring lying down and predilection for sitting, and insufficient exercise. As people reach middle and older age, their spleen-stomach movement and transformation function gradually declines and their metabolism of fats, sweets, and thick flavors gradually becomes weaker. The finest essence of water and grains is not able to be transformed, engendered, transported, and spread. Instead, pasty fat, phlegm, and dampness lodge internally. Based on this theory of obesity, the body acupuncture points in the above protocol were selected in order to regulate and rectify the spleen-stomach functions of movement and transformation as well as to drain excessive stomach fire, free the flow and discharge the large intestine, rectify the qi and fortify the spleen, dispel phlegm and disinhibit dampness, warm the kidneys and invigorate yang, course the liver and rectify the qi, clear and downbear liver yang. The ear points were selected to regulate and rectify the function of the viscera and bowels, decrease hunger and promote a feeling of satiety. In terms of dietary therapy, for breakfast, the patients mainly ate egg whites. For lunch they ate lots of vegetables and a little grains. For dinner, they ate lots of vegetables and a little egg whites. During this study, patient's diets were not excessively regulated so as to avoid hypoglycemic syncope or disturbances in work or study. In general, the patients that exercised the most or were the most active got the best outcomes.

7. In issue #2, 2004 of *Ji Lin Zhong Yi Yao* (*Jilin Chinese Medicine & Medicinals*), Zhang Hong-ying published an article titled, "The Treatment of 46 Cases of Simple Obesity with Acupuncture as the Main Treatment," on page 34 of that journal.

Cohort description
All 46 cases were seen as outpatients in the acupuncture-moxibustion department of the author's hospital in Tianjin and all met published criteria for simple obesity. Among these, 40 were females and six were males. The youngest was 16 and the oldest was 45 years old. The heaviest patient weighed 107 kilograms and the lightest weighed 62 kilograms. The shortest course of disease was one year and the longest was 20 years, with an average disease duration of 6.7 years.

Treatment method
Patients were divided according to three patterns: 1) stomach and intestinal replete heat, 2) spleen vacuity with damp obstruction, and 3) liver qi depression and binding. The points chosen (for all patients) consisted of:

Zhong Wan (CV 12)
Shui Fen (CV 9)
Tian Shu (St 25)
Hua Rou Men (St 24)
Wai Ling (St 26)
Bi Guan (St 31)
Liang Qiu (St 34)
Zu San Li (St 36)
Yin Ling Quan (Sp 9)

For those who presented with stomach and intestinal replete heat, *Qu Chi* (LI 11) and *Shang Ju Xu* (St 37) were added. For those who presented with spleen vacuity with damp obstruction, *Feng Long* (St 40), *San Yin Jiao* (Sp 6), and *Gong Sun* (Sp 4) were added. For those who presented with liver qi depression and binding, *Tai Chong* (Liv 3) and *Zhi Gou* (TB 6) were added. Treatment was given once every other day with a needle retention of 20 minutes each time. Twenty such treatments equaled one course of therapy, and outcomes were analyzed after one such course.

Patients were also orally administered a weight-loss tea. This consisted of:

He Ye (Folium Nelumbinis), 10g
Jue Ming Zi (Semen Cassiae), 10g
Shan Zha (Fructus Crataegi), 12g
Ze Xie (Rhizoma Alismatis), 10g

One packet of these medicinals was decocted into water and drunk as a tea for two days.

In terms of dietary therapy, patients were instructed to reduce their consumption of fatty, sweet, thick-flavored foods and to only eat three times per day, breakfast, lunch, and dinner. These meals were to be taken at fixed times every day and were to consist of fixed amounts. For breakfast, patients in this study were allowed 1-2 eggs, 50 grams of cereal, or 250ml of milk. For lunch, they were allowed 50 grams of cereals, 100 grams of lean meat, and a suitable amount of clear, bland, stir-fried vegetables to the point of feeling full. For dinner, they were allowed to have only 100 grams of clear, bland, stir-fried vegetables.

Exercise consisted of 30-60 minutes of aerobic exercise per day keeping their heart rate between 120-130 beats per minute. Any feeling of fatigue or exhaustion gradually disappeared within 10-20 minutes after stopping the exercise.

Study outcomes
A marked effect was defined as a reduction in body weight of five kilograms or more. Some effect meant that there was a reduction in weight of three kilos or more, and no effect meant that patients lost only two kilos or less. Based on these criteria, 30 out of 46 patients (65.2%) registered a marked effect, 12 patients (26.1%) got some effect, and only four patients (8.7%) got no effect. Therefore, the total effectiveness rate was published as 91.3%.

8. On pages 134-135 in issue #3, 2006 of the *Zhe Jiang Zhong Yi Za Zhi (Zhejiang Journal of Chinese Medicine)*, Xu Bing-guo & Liu Zhi-cheng published an article titled, "Acupuncture's Influence on the Levels of Nitric Oxide & Nitric Oxide Synthase in Patients with Obesity & Hypertension."

Cohort description
There were 30 patients enrolled in this study, all of whom met the diagnostic criteria for simple obesity as well as the 1999 criteria for hypertension set forth in *Zhong Guo Gao Xue Ya Fang Zhi Zhi Nan (A Guide to the Prevention & Treatment of Hypertension in China)*. Twenty-five of these patients were female and five were male. These patients' ages ranged from 22 to 72 years, with a mean age of 45.2 ≥ 10.1 years. Their course of disease ranged from 0.5-30 years, with a mean duration of 10.8 ≥ 7.5 years. In addition, there was another group of 25 normal, healthy patients which served as a comparison. In terms of sex and age, these two groups were statistically comparable.

Treatment method
The patients in the treatment group were divided into four Chinese medical patterns and then received different ear and body acupuncture protocols depending on their presenting pattern.

1. Liver fire hyperactivity & exuberance pattern (10 cases)

In order to clear the liver and drain fire, the ear points chosen were:

1. Liver   3. Triple Burner
2. Gallbladder   4. Sympathetic

The body points chosen consisted of:

Feng Chi (GB 20)
Gan Shu (Bl 18)
Qu Chi (LI 11)
Yang Ling Quan (GB 34)
Tai Chong (Liv 3)
Xing Jian (Liv 2)

2. Yin vacuity-yang hyperactivity pattern (six cases)

In order to enrich yin and subdue yang, the ear points chosen were:

1. Liver   3. Internal Secretion (Endocrine)
2. Kidney   4. Sympathetic

The body points chosen were:

Feng Chi (GB 20)
Gan Shu (Bl 18)
Shen Shu (Bl 23)
San Yin Jiao (Sp 6)
Tai Chong (Liv 3)
Tai Xi (Ki 3)

3. Yin & yang dual vacuity pattern (three cases)

In order to regulate and supplement yin and yang, the ear points chosen were:

1. Liver   3. Endocrine
2. Kidney   4. Shen Men

The body points chosen consisted of:

Gan Shu (Bl 18)
Shen Shu (Bl 23)
Ming Men (GV 4)
Guan Yuan (CV 4)
San Yin Jiao (Sp 6)
Tai Xi (Ki 3)

4. Phlegm dampness congestion & exuberance pattern (11 cases)

In order to transform phlegm and dispel dampness, the ear points chosen were:

1. Spleen   3. Endocrine
2. Stomach   4. Triple Burner

The body points chosen were:

Pi Shu (Bl 20)
Zhong Wan (CV 12)
Yin Ling Quan (Sp 9)
Zu San Li (St 36)
Feng Long (St 40)
Tai Bai (Sp 3)

Wang Bu Liu Xing (Semen Vaccariae) seeds were taped over the ear points with adhesive and each point was stimulated three times per day with finger pressure. Each point was stimulated for 1-2 minutes per time. The points were switched from ear to ear every other day. Body acupuncture was administered once every other day, with the needles retained for 30 minutes each time. After obtaining the qi, draining hand technique was applied to those who were mostly replete, and supplementing hand technique was applied to those who were mainly vacuous. One month equaled one course of treatment, and three courses were administered.

Study outcomes
Patients' body mass index (BMI), weight, and circumference were measured before and after treatment. Circumference was measured at the chest, waist, upper arm, and thigh. Skin thickness was also measured before and after treatment at the back of the elbow, the axilla of the shoulder, and the abdomen as were NO and NOS. Based on these measurements, 10 cases (33.3%) were judged to have experienced a marked effect, 14 cases (46.67%) got some effect, and six cases (20%) got no effect. Therefore, the total effectiveness was stated as 80%. The following table shows the differences in NO and NOS before and after treatment as well as the differences in these two values between the healthy comparison group and the diseased patients.

Criteria	Normal group (25)	Patients before treatment (30)	Patients after treatment (30)
NO (umol/L)	76.10 ± 17.10	55.384 ± 19.526	89.391 ± 33.249
NOS (U/mL)	37.84 ± 3.63	31.659 ± 3.281	35.510 ± 3.289

This table shows that NO levels in the obese patients were significantly lower than in the healthy comparison group before treatment and that these levels significantly increased after treatment. Similarly, NOS levels were lower in the obese patients than the healthy group and also increased after treatment. However, even after treatment, these levels were still not as high as in the comparison group. Based on these outcomes, it appears that the combination of ear and body acupuncture is effective for treating obesity, decreasing blood pressure, and normalizing NO and NOS levels in the body.

9. On pages 220-221 of issue #4, 2006 of the *Zhe Jiang Zhong Yi Za Zhi (Zhejiang Journal of Chinese Medicine)*, Qiu Xiao-ling et al. published an article titled, "Clinical Observations on the Acupuncture Treatment of Simple Obesity & Hyperlipoproteinemia."

Cohort description
Altogether, there were 90 patients enrolled in this two-wing comparison study. Among these 90 patients, there were 72 females and eight males 25-64 years of age with a disease duration of from 1-27 years. These patients were randomly divided into two groups of 45 patients each which were judged statistically comparable in terms of age, sex, obesity level, blood lipid levels, and disease duration. One of these groups received acupuncture plus electroacupuncture and the other received acupuncture plus hand stimulation. All had a body mass index (BMI) of 25 points or more. In addition, all had total cholesterol (TC) of 6.0mmol/L or more, triglycerides (TG) of 1.70mmol/L, high density lipids (HDL-C) of 1.04mmol/L or less if male, or low density lipids (LDL-C) of 1.17mmol/L or more if female. Exclusion criteria included hypothyroidism, liver disease, kidney disease, diabetes, or drug therapy causing high cholesterol.

Treatment method
The basic acupuncture points used on all members of both groups consisted of:

Zhong Wan (CV 12)
Xia Wan (CV 10)
Shui Fen (CV 9)
Qi Hai (CV 6)
Guan Yuan (CV 4)
Hua Rou Men (St 24)
Wai Ling (St 26)
Da Heng (Sp 15)
Tian Shu (St 25)
Qu Chi (LI 11)
Zu San Li (St 36)
San Yin Jiao (Sp 6)

If there was spleen vacuity with damp obstruction, *Yin Ling Quan* (Sp 9), *Gong Sun* (Sp 4), and *Feng Long* (St 40) were added. If there was stomach and intestinal replete heat, *Zhi Gou* (TB 6) and *Gui Lai* (St 29) were added. If there was qi stagnation and blood stasis, *Xue Hai* (Sp 10) and *Tai Chong* (Liv 3) were added. If there was spleen-kidney yang vacuity, *Pi Shu* (Bl 20), *Shen Shu* (Bl 23), and *Tai Xi* (Ki 3) were added.

Members of group A received acupuncture plus electro-acupuncture stimulation. Fine needles 0.25 x 50 millimeters were inserted into the above points and then manipulated with even supplementing-even draining technique. In addition, after obtaining the qi, *Qu Chi* and *Zu San Li* were stimulated electrically using a G-6805 electro-acupuncture device with a high frequency continuous wave. The needles were retained for 30 minutes. Members of group B were also needled with the same size fine needles. After obtaining the qi, those manifesting repletion patterns were treated with twisting and twirling draining hand technique, while those manifesting vacuity patterns were treated with twisting and twirling supplementing hand technique. The needles at *Qu Chi* and *Zu San Li* were manipulated every 10 minutes, with the needles also being retained for 30 minutes. Both groups were thus treated one time every other day, with 10 treatments equaling one course and three courses being given.

Study outcomes
Cure was defined as a complete disappearance of clinical symptoms and less than 20% body fat in men and less than 30% in women or a BMI within normal parameters. A marked effect was defined as a basic disappearance of clinical symptoms with a reduction of weight of five kilograms or more or a reduction in percentage of body fat of 5% or more. Improvement meant that there was an improvement in clinical symptoms and a loss of two kilograms of weight or more or a reduction in body fat of 1% or more. No effect meant that there was no obvious improvement in clinical symptoms and any loss of weight was less than two kilograms and any reduction in body fat was less than 1%. The following table shows the outcomes based on these criteria.

Group	Cured	Marked effect	Improvement	No effect	Total effect
A	5	15	16	9	80.0%
B	8	19	14	4	91.1%

These outcomes suggest that hand stimulation is superior than electrical stimulation in weight-loss acupuncture, at least at *Qu Chi* and *Zu San Li*. In addition, after treatment, group B had a greater mean loss of weight, a lower mean percentage of body fat, and a lower mean BMI score than did group A. Prior to treatment there was no significant statistical differences in the mean scores between these two groups. Similarly, after treatment group B had significantly lower mean TC and significantly higher mean HDL-C than group A.

Discussion
According to the Chinese authors of this study, obesity is mainly due to a former heaven natural endowment insufficiency combined with unregulated diet, prolonged sitting and scanty exercise, and loss of regulation of the mind and emotions resulting in loss of regulation in the qi and blood, yin and yang, and function of the viscera and bowels. If the triple burner original qi is insufficient, this leads to water dampness, phlegm turbidity, and greasy fat congesting and becoming exuberant in the interior of the body. This condition is mainly located in the three viscera of the liver, spleen, and kidneys. However, it is especially centered in the spleen and kidneys. If the spleen loses its fortification and movement, the movement and transformation of water dampness and the finest essence of water and grains will lose their normalcy, resulting in the internal engenderment of phlegm turbidity or phlegm dampness. Therefore, the authors believe that acupuncture for obesity and high cholesterol should mainly regulate and rectify the spleen and stomach and supplement the kidneys assisted by quickening the blood and transforming stasis, coursing the liver and disinhibiting the gallbladder. Within the above protocol, they say that *Zhong Wan, Xia Wan, Shui Fen, Hua Rou Men, Wai Ling, Tian Shu, Da Heng, Zu San Li, Qi Hai*, and *Guan Yuan* fortify and move the spleen and stomach, transform dampness and disinhibit water, disperse and eliminate accumulation and stagnation, warm the kidneys and invigorate yang. In addition, *Yin Ling Quan, Gong Sun*, and *Feng Long* strengthen the fortification of the spleen, the transformation of dampness, and the elimination of phlegm, while *Zhi Gou* and *Gui Lai* drain stomach fire and free the flow and regulate the bowel qi. *Xue Hai* and *Tai Chong* move the qi and quicken the blood, and *Pi Shu, Shen Shu*, and *Tai Xi* boost the source of fire.

10. On page 72 of issue #2, 2006 of the *Zhe Jiang Zhong Yi Za Zhi (Zhejiang Journal of Chinese Medicine)*, Wu Wei-ping published an article titled, "The Treatment of 80 Cases of Simple Obesity with Point Catgut Embedding."

Cohort description
All 80 patients in this clinical trial were seen as outpatients. Among them,

there were 18 males and 62 females with an average age of 28.5 years. The diagnosis of obesity was based on body mass index (BMI). All patients in this study had a BMI of 23.10 or greater. The highest BMI was 35.20 and the lowest was 23.10. The average was 25.19. Patients with obesity secondary to some neuro-endocrinological disorder were excluded from this study.

Treatment method
The points selected for treatment in this trial included:

Tian Shu (St 25)
Da Heng (Sp 15)
Zhong Wan (CV 12)
Qi Hai (CV 6)
Liang Qiu (St 34)
Shang Ju Xu (St 37)
Zu San Li (St 36)
Feng Long (St 40)

After disinfection, 00 gauge catgut was embedded in each of these points. This was done three times once every 20 days. During the course of treatment, patients were supposed to control their diet by lowering the amount of processed foods, fatty foods, and carbohydrates but increasing their protein. Patients were counseled against eating an excessive amount of fats and sugar but to eat plenty of fresh vegetables, dairy products, eggs, and seafood.

Study outcomes
Marked effect was defined as a loss of weight of five kilograms or more. Some effect was defined as a loss of weight of 2.5 kilograms. No effect meant that the patient did not lose at least 2.5 kilograms of weight. Based on these criteria, 45 cases (56.2%) got a marked effect, 31 cases (38.8%) got some effect, and four cases (5%) got no effect. Therefore, the total effectiveness rate was listed as 95%.

Discussion
According to Dr. Wu, accompanying symptoms, such as acne, chronic fatigue syndrome, constipation, menstrual irregularities, hypertension, high cholesterol, diabetes, and fatty liver all also improved during this trial.

11. On page 97 of issue #1, 2006 of the *Shi Yong Zhong Yi Nei Ke Za Zhi* (*Journal of Practical Chinese Medicine Internal Medicine*), Wang Su-ling published an article titled, "The Treatment of 100 Cases of Obesity with Point Catgut Embedding."

Cohort description

All 100 patients in this study were seen as outpatients. Among them, there were 36 males and 64 females 18-75 years old who had been overweight for from two to 16 years. Obesity was based on each patient's body mass index (BMI).

Treatment method

The points chosen for treatment included:

Zhong Wan (CV 12)
Shang Wan (CV 13)
Tian Shu (St 25)
Qi Hai (CV 6)
Pi Shu (Bl 20)
Wei Shu (Bl 21)

After disinfection, one centimeter long pieces of catgut were embedded in each of the above points. Two weeks later, these were replaced. Five such treatments equaled one course of therapy. During this treatment, the patients were also asked to reduce their intake of processed foods, fatty foods, and carbohydrates but to increase their protein. They were told to restrict their intake of fatty foods and sugar but to eat lots of fresh vegetables, dairy products, eggs, and high protein foods.

Study outcomes

Cure was defined as the attainment of ideal BMI. Marked effect was defined as a loss of weight of five kilograms. Some effect meant a loss of weight of three kilograms, while no effect meant that any weight lost was less than three kilograms. Based on these criteria, 20 cases were cured, 38 experienced a marked effect, 30 got some effect, and 12 got no effect, for a total effectiveness rate of 88%.

Discussion

According to Dr. Wang, the above therapy was intended to regulate and rectify the spleen and stomach, upbear the clear and downbear the turbid.

12. On page 25 of issue #4, 2005 of the *Jiang Xi Zhong Yao Yue (Jiangxi Review of Chinese Medicine)*, Li Shu-xia published an article titled "The Treatment of Pediatric Simple Obesity with *Wen Dan Tang* (Warm the Gallbladder Decoction)."

Cohort description
Of the 30 cases of pediatric obesity enrolled in this study, 19 were male and 11 were female and all were between 7-13 years old. The children had an accumulation of fat in their upper arms, buttocks, abdomen, etc. Each of these cases was classified as either mild, medium, or severe obesity. Patients who had mild obesity had a body weight 20% above normal, medium obesity meant being 30-50% above normal body weight, and severe obesity meant a body weight more than 50% above normal. Endocrine function was tested to differentiate simple obesity from obesity due to endocrine dysfunction.

Treatment method
All patients enrolled in this clinical trial were administered the following basic Chinese herbal formula:

Ban Xia (Rhizoma Pinelliae), 6g
Zhu Ru (Caulis Bambusae In Taeniis), 6g
Zhi Shi (Fructus Immaturus Aurantii), 6g
Fu Ling (Poria), 6g
Huang Lian (Rhizoma Coptidis), 3g
Da Huang (Radix Et Rhizoma Rhei), 3-6g
Chen Pi (Pericarpium Citri Reticulatae), 9g
Sheng Jiang (uncooked Rhizoma Zingiberis), 3 slices
Da Zao (Fructus Jujubae), 2 pieces

If there was qi vacuity with lack of strength, *Huang Lian* and *Zhu Ru* were subtracted and six grams of *Lian Qiao* (Fructus Forsythiae), 12 grams of *Huang Qi* (Radix Astragali), and six grams each of *Dang Shen* (Radix Codonopsitis) and *Bai Zhu* (Rhizoma Atractylodis Macrocephalae) were added. If there was slimy tongue fur and greater dampness, *Gua Lou* (Fructus Trichosanthis), *Cang Zhu* (Rhizoma Atractylodis), and *Hou Po* (Cortex Magnoliae Officinalis) were added. One packet of the above medicinals were decocted in water and administered per day. Ten days equaled one course of treatment, and a five day interval was allowed between each course of treatment.

Study outcomes

Of the 30 children who were initially enrolled in this study, two would not take the Chinese medicinals. However, there was a reduction in the severity of the obesity in all the other 28 children after 2-3 courses of treatment. During treatment, the patients reduced their weight by 3-6 kilograms. The herbal formula was combined with physical exercise and a regulated diet. A follow-up visit showed the weight loss was maintained for six months.

Discussion

In the above formula, *Dang Shen, Fu Ling,* and *Chen Pi* fortify the spleen and supplement the kidneys in order to assist the bodily function of transportation and to dispel evils. *Ban Xia, Zhu Ru, Zhi Shi,* and *Huang Lian* transform phlegm and eliminate dampness. *Da Huang* eliminates phlegm-dampness and flushes the intestines and stomach. This medicinal "pushes (out) the old, resulting in new," calms and harmonizes the five viscera, and, when combined with medicinals that fortify the spleen and supplement the kidneys, is not excessively attacking. The author says this formula is reliable in achieving good results in treating simple obesity due to its ability to simultaneously fortify the spleen and supplement the kidneys, flush phlegm and eliminate dampness.

13. On pages 53-54 of issue #2, 2006 of *Shan Xi Zhong Yi (Shanxi Chinese Medicine),* Wang Xiao-ying et al. published an article titled, "Clinical Observations of the Treatment of Simple Obesity with *Hua Tan Jian Fei Tang* (Transform Phlegm & Reduce Fat Decoction)."

Cohort description

Altogether, there were 90 overweight patients enrolled in this study, 32 males and 58 females aged 14-55 years, with an average age of 43.61 years. These patients weighed between 61.5-108.0 kilograms, with an average weight of 78-79 kilograms. Their body mass index (BMI) ranged from 24.9-27.9kg/m² in 69 cases and was over 28.0kg/m² in 21 cases. Eighteen cases had accompanying fatty livers, 36 had high cholesterol, six had high blood pressure, and nine had coronary heart disease. Excluded from this study were those with endocrine disorders resulting in obesity, those with serious heart, cerebral, liver, or kidney disease, and those with a BMI less than 24.0.

Treatment method

Hua Tan Jian Fei Tang (Transform Phlegm & Reduce Fat Decoction) consisted of:

Fu Ling (Poria), 5-10g
Gui Zhi (Ramulus Cinnamomi), 5-10g
Bai Zhu (Rhizoma Atractylodis Macrocephalae), 10-15g
Shan Zha (Fructus Crataegi), 15-30g
Da Huang (Radix Et Rhizoma Rhei), 6-10g
Ze Xie (Rhizoma Alismatis), 6-10g
Gan Cao (Radix Glycyrrhizae), 3-6g

    One packet of these medicinals was decocted in water and administered warm per day, with three months continuous treatment equaling one course. A one week rest was allowed in between each successive month. While taking these medicinals, patients were counseled to avoid high fat, high sugar, and high salt foods and drinks. On top of their basic daily diet, they were asked to eat one egg per day and one glass of milk but to continue exercising the same as before initiating treatment. Their weight, waist circumference, and blood lipids were measured once each month.

Study outcomes
The following table shows the mean differences in weight, waist size, buttock size, and BMI from before to after treatment.

Time	Weight (kg)	Waist size (cm)	Buttock size (cm)	BMI
Before Treatment	78.9 ± 10.8	90.50 ± 8.69	99.30 ± 5.47	28.81 ± 3.35
After Treatment	75.1 ± 10.1	84.97 ± 8.47	97.50 ± 6.52	27.44 ± 3.38

Discussion
Within this formula, *Fu Ling, Bai Zhu,* and *Gui Zhi* warm and transform the yin evils of phlegm and dampness. *Shan Zha* arouses the spleen and disperses food, quickens the blood and scatters stasis. *Da Huang* quickens the blood and scatters stasis, scours and washes clean the intestines and stomach. *Ze Xie* combined with *Bai Zhu* fortifies the spleen and disinhibits dampness. *Gan Cao* then regulates and harmonizes all the other medicinals in the formula as well as fortifies the spleen and harmonizes the center. When all these medicinals are used together, they warm and transform phlegm and stasis, reduce fat and decrease obesity.

14. On page 36 of issue #3, 2006 of *Shan Xi Zhong Yi (Shanxi Chinese Medicine)*, Chen Luan-xiang published an article titled, "Clinical Observations on the Treatment of Simple Obesity with Acupuncture."

Cohort description

There were 75 patients enrolled in this study, 62 females and 13 males aged 28-59 years. All were 20% or more above their ideal body weight with a BMI of 26 or more. All these patients also had abnormalities in their total cholesterol (TC), triglycerides (TG), high density lipids (HDL), low density lipids (LDL), and fasting blood glucose (FBG).

Treatment method

The points chosen from consisted of:

Zu San Li (St 36)
Nei Ting (St 44)
Tian Shu (St 25)
Qi Hai (CV 6)
Guan Yuan (CV 4)
Zhong Wan (CV 12)
Shang Ju Xu (St 37)
Xia Ju Xu (St 39)
Xing Jian (Liv 2)

Plus other points on the foot yang ming stomach channel. For instance, if there was spleen vacuity with damp obstruction, *Guan Men* (St 22), *Tai Yi* (St 23), *Zu San Li* (St 36), and *Feng Long* (St 40) were chosen. If there was stomach heat with damp obstruction, *Zu San Li* (St 36), *Shang Ju Xu* (St 37), *Xia Ju Xu* (St 39), and *Nei Ting* (St 44) were chosen. If there was constipation, *Tian Shu* (St 25), *Shui Dao* (St 28), *Zu San Li* (St 36), *Shang Ju Xu* (St 37), and *Xia Ju Xu* (St 39) were chosen. If there was edema, *Feng Long* (St 40), *Yang Ling Quan* (GB 34), *San Yin Jiao* (Sp 6), and *Shui Dao* (St 28) were chosen. If heat was heavy, *Qu Chi* (LI 11) and *He Gu* (LI 4) were chosen. If the patient had a hard time losing weight, *Tian Shu* (St 25), *Hua Rou Men* (St 24), *Zu San Li* (St 36), and *Feng Long* (St 40) were chosen. These points were needled once per day for five days. Then a two day rest was allowed before another five day course was given. Altogether, four such courses were administered.

Study outcomes

Study outcomes were expressed as changes in mean values from before to after treatment as shown by the following table.

	Weight (kg)	TC (mmol/L)	HDL (mmol/L)	LDL (mmol/L)	TG (mmol/L)	FBG (mmol/L)
Before Treatment	74.31 ± 8.89	5.46 ± 0.99	1.21 ± 0.21	3.72 ± 1.00	2.26 ± 1.02	5.70 ± 0.86
After Treatment	71.41 ± 9.0	4.43 ± 0.95	1.26 ± 0.17	2.64 ± 0.91	1.39 ± 0.56	4.90 ± 0.61

Therefore, there was a statistically significant mean change towards the better in all these parameters from before to after treatment ($P < 0.01$).

15. On page 13 of issue #3, 2006 of *Fu Jian Zhong Yi Yao (Fujian Chinese Medicine & Medicinals)*, Tai Yong-jun et al. published an article titled, "The Treatment of 108 Cases of Simple Obesity with Acupuncture Combined with Ear Pressure."

Cohort description
Altogether, there were 158 patients enrolled in this two-wing comparison study, 130 females and 28 males aged 17-65, with a mean age of 45 ± 0.2 years. The course of disease had lasted from 1-20 years, with a mean duration of 5.5 ± 0.2 years. Sixty-eight patients were grossly obese, 58 were slightly obese, and 23 were moderately obese. The definition of obesity was being more than 20% over one's ideal body weight, with fat making up 30% or more of a woman's total mass and 25% or more of a man's. These patients were randomly divided into two groups: a treatment group of 108 and a comparison group of 50. In terms of age, sex, duration, and degree of obesity, these two groups were comparable for the purposes of this study.

Treatment method
All members of the treatment group were discriminated into one of the following patterns: spleen vacuity with damp obstruction, stomach heat with damp obstruction, liver depression qi stagnation, spleen-kidney dual vacuity, or yin vacuity with internal heat. The main body points for all these patients included:

Zhong Wan (CV 12)
Xia Wan (CV 10)
Qi Hai (CV 6)
Tian Shu (St 25)
Da Heng (Sp 15)
Fu Jie (Sp 14)
Feng Long (St 40)

If there was spleen vacuity with damp obstruction, *San Yin Jiao* (Sp 6), *Gong Sun* (Sp 4), and *Zu San Li* (St 36) were added. If there was stomach heat with damp obstruction, *Qu Chi* (LI 11), *He Gu* (LI 4), *Nei Ting* (St 44), and *Liang Qiu* (St 34) were added. If there was liver depression qi stagnation, *Shan Zhong* (CV 17), *Qi Men* (Liv 14), *Yang Ling Quan* (GB 34), and *Tai Chong* (Liv 3) were added. If there was spleen-kidney dual vacuity, *Guan Yuan* (CV 4), *Zu San Li* (St 36), *San Yin Jiao* (Sp 6), and *Tai Xi* (Ki 3) were added. If there was yin vacuity with internal heat, *Shang Wan* (CV 13), *Shou San Li* (LI 10), *Zu San Li* (St 36), and *Xia Ju Xu* (St 39) were added. If there was constipation, *Zhi Gou* (TB 6) was added. If there was edema, *Shui Fen* (CV 9), *Yang Ling Quan* (GB 34), and *San Yin Jiao* (Sp 6) were added. If there was menstrual irregularity, *Dai Mai* (GB 26), *Xue Hai* (Sp 10), *Di Ji* (Sp 8), and *San Yin Jiao* (Sp 6) were added. Electro-acupuncture was administered using a 6805 electro-acupuncture machine. Treatment was given once per day for 45 minutes. After three days, a one day rest was allowed. Thirty such treatments equaled one course of therapy. After one course of treatment, a one month rest was allowed before starting a second course.

Ear pressure consisted of stimulating the following points:

1. Hunger	5. Shen Men
2. Endocrine	6. Liver
3. Thyroid	7. Spleen
4. Sympathetic	8. Kidney

A seed of *Wang Bu Liu Xing* (Semen Vaccariae) was fixed bilaterally to each point for 3-4 days. Each day, the patient was instructed to press these points softly for 15 minutes.

All members of the comparison group only received the same ear pressure point treatment.

Study outcomes
Marked effect was defined as a weight loss of five kilograms or more or five percent of body weight plus a decrease in percentage of body fat of five percent and a reduction in waist circumference of eight centimeters. Some effect was defined as a loss of three kilograms or more or a loss of three percent body weight plus a decrease in body fat of three percent and a decrease in waist circumference of four centimeters. No effect meant that neither of these criteria were met. The following table shows the outcomes based on these criteria.

Group	Marked effect	Some effect	No effect	Total effect
Treatment	48 (44.1%)	54 (50.0%)	6 (5.9%)	94.1%
Comparison	14 (28.0%)	26 (52.0%)	10 (20.0%)	80.0%

Therefore, it was concluded that electro-acupuncture plus ear pressure was significantly more effective than ear pressure alone.

16. On page 18 of issue #3, 2006 of *Fu Jian Zhong Yi Yao (Fujian Chinese Medicine & Medicinals)*, Wang Feng-yin et al. published an article titled, "The Treatment of 580 Cases of Simple Obesity with Acupuncture Combined with Ear Point Pressure."

Cohort description
All 580 patients in this study were female, and their ages ranged from 16-50 years, with an average age of 38.5. Their course of disease had lasted from 0.5-15 years, with an average disease duration of six years. One hundred sixty-two women were unmarried and 418 were married. The 1987 National Symposium on Integrated Chinese-Western Medicine criteria for obesity were used. Slight obesity meant that the patient was 20% above her ideal body mass index (BMI), moderate obesity meant she was 30% over her ideal BMI, and gross obesity meant that she was 50% over her ideal BMI. Therefore, 105 of these women were slightly obese, 432 were moderately obese, and 43 were grossly obese. Patients with organic disease of the heart, liver, and kidneys were excluded from this study.

Treatment method
The main acupoints chosen on the abdomen included:

Tian Shu (St 25)
Da Heng (Sp 15)
Qi Hai (CV 6)
Hua Rou Men (St 24)
Shang Wan (CV 13)
Zhong Wan (CV 12)

The main points on the upper extremities included:

Qu Chi (LI 11)
Zhi Gou (TB 6)

The main points on the lower extremities included:

Liang Qiu (St 34)
Feng Shi (GB 31)

If there was spleen vacuity with damp obstruction, *Zu San Li* (St 36), *San Yin Jiao* (Sp 6), *Yin Ling Quan* (Sp 9), and *Gong Sun* (Sp 4) were added. If there was stomach heat with damp obstruction, *He Gu* (LI 4), *Qu Chi* (LI 11), *Feng Long* (St 40), and *Nei Ting* (St 44) were added. If there was spleen-kidney dual vacuity, *Guan Yuan* (CV 4), *Zu San Li* (St 36), and *San Yin Jiao* (Sp 6) were added. If there was yin vacuity with internal heat, *Nei Guan* (Per 6), *San Yin Jiao* (Sp 6), and *Tai Xi* (Ki 3) were added. Thirty-five gauge needles were used. After obtaining the qi, draining hand technique was used and the needles were retained for 30 minutes. During this time, the needles were stimulated 2-3 times. One treatment was given per day for three days and then a one day rest was allowed. Fifteen treatments equaled one course, and a one week rest was allowed between successive courses.

Ear points stimulated included:

1. Shen Men	5. Large Intestine
2. Endocrine	6. Kidney
3. Triple Burner	7. Hunger
4. Stomach	8. Thirst

Seeds of *Wang Bu Liu Xing* (Semen Vaccariae) were affixed to each point and pressed until the patient felt soreness, distention, and/or a hot feeling. The points were pressed for 3-5 minutes once each day. Points were only stimulated on one ear at a time. Every three days the ears were switched one time. Ten times or switches equaled one course of treatment.

Study outcomes
Cure meant that, after a single course of treatment, the patient's weight and waist circumference were within normal parameters. Marked effect meant that the patient lost five kilograms or more. Some effect meant that she lost three kilograms or more, and no effect meant that she did not lose three kilograms. Based on these criteria, 328 women (56.6%) were cured, 179 (30.9%) got a marked effect, 60 (10.3%) got some effect, and 13 (2.2%) got no effect. Therefore, the total effectiveness rate was stated as 97.8%. Further, the best results (100%) were achieved in those who were only slightly obese, while the worst results (76.4%) were seen in those who were grossly obese.

Healthy Eating 6

R ight diet is so important to good health that at my center for Chinese medicine (Aiyana Acupuncture & Chinese Herbs in NYC), every patient I see receives dietary counseling for health maintenance and to treat their personally presenting Chinese medical patterns. The majority of tips and suggestions in this chapter can be used by anyone who seeks a healthier eating style regardless of a need for weight loss.

Right diet does not have to be hard

Usually patients declare their intent to diet with an anguished moan, but healthy eating and weight loss do not have to be a chore. It is much easier to lose weight and keep it off when the patient shifts their perception about dieting. The most important shift is the realization that dieting does not have to be about deprivation. A dieter does not have to live on bland salads, eating only soups or prepackaged diet plan meals, or go on controversial induction or crash diets to lose weight. In fact, Chinese medicine advises quite the opposite. We advise balance, not deprivation, as the best way to achieve and maintain a healthy body. Depriving the body of food deprives the body of much needed qi, blood, and body fluids.

> We advise balance, not deprivation, as the best way to achieve and maintain a healthy body. Depriving the body of food deprives the body of much needed qi, blood, and body fluids.

Modern nutritional research has revealed that many of the foods we once thought were unhealthy and led to weight gain are actually healthy. In fact,

even some fats, like olive oil, contribute to good health by lowering cholesterol. However, most modern convenience foods, popular since the early
1960s, have proven extremely unhealthy. This includes processed foods, sugary snacks, many frozen, boxed, and canned foods, and, of course, fast food.
However, in recent years, the consumer demand for healthier grocery choices
has prompted food manufacturers to adjust to this demand. Now, many
manufacturers specialize in whole, healthy, and/or organic foods, and major
brands have produced new lines of healthy, whole grain breads and pastas to
meet consumer demand. Restaurants are also following this trend by adding
healthy menu items.

Chinese dietary therapy

Chinese dietary therapy and its balancing techniques usually require simple,
natural changes as opposed to many of the extreme or hard-to-follow diets
popular in America. In Chinese medicine, a balanced style of eating means balance of the yin and yang. Yin foods help supplement yin fluids (*yin ye* 阴液)
and build physical substance. Yang foods help supplement the yang qi (*yang
qi* 阳气) and promote metabolic function. One of the main determinants of
whether a food is yin or yang in Chinese medicine is the food's thermal nature.
The five thermal natures of foods in Chinese medicine are hot, warm, neutral,
cool, and cold. (See Appendix B for a list of foods broken down according to
these temperatures.) If the patient exhibits a yang vacuity pattern, she or he
should eat more yang-supplementing foods until the pattern of disharmony is
balanced. Once the therapeutic goal is achieved, the practitioner should
instruct the patient to commence with an energetically balanced eating style
based on the constitutional propensity of the patient. If she or he has a yin
constitution, balance will be maintained by eating more warming rather than
cooling foods in proportion to the disharmony. She or he should eat both
warming and cooling foods but balance more toward the warm side to warm
the cool, yin constitution. In other words, balance is based on the individual's
overall Chinese medical propensity.

For example, a constitutionally cool patient should be advised to balance
diet toward the warm. For breakfast, this may mean eating cooked oatmeal
with cinnamon and dates (warm). For lunch, this may mean eating a turkey
(warm) sandwich on whole wheat bread (cool), spread with basil pesto
(warm) with lettuce (cool) and a cup of vegetable soup (warm). For dinner,
the patient might eat coconut grilled shrimp (warm) and jasmine rice (neutral) with spinach (cool) sautéed in garlic (hot) and olive oil (warm).

Chinese medicine uses foods therapeutically, just like herbs, to balance disharmony. In fact, there is a saying, "Food and medicine share a common source." Chinese medicine recommends that therapeutic food be taken only throughout the duration of illness. If the patient has a cold condition and eats mainly hot foods longer than therapeutically indicated, her condition can change to a heat condition. Once the disharmony is balanced, diet alterations can be made according to the season. In winter, the patient should eat more warming foods, and in summer, she should eat more cooling foods. During damp times of year or for patients who live in overly damp climates, Chinese medical practitioners should encourage the increased consumption of warming and dampness-drying foods.

Overconsumption of cool or cold foods (including raw fruits and vegetables) damage spleen and stomach yang qi leading to cold and dampness. Cold damp stagnation can then lead to weight gain. According to Chinese medicine, "The spleen is averse to cold," and, "The spleen is averse to dampness." This means that cold and damp foods harm the spleen qi. The spleen is the vital organ for the movement and transformation of food and drink. It transforms the food and drink into qi, blood, and body fluids and transports these to the other organs and tissues so that they can properly perform their functions in preserving physiological balance and harmony. When organ systems do not receive enough qi, the disharmony caused by that deprivation can lead to disease. overconsumption of cold foods may also injure the kidney qi. Kidney vacuity with water spilling over is a yang vacuity failing to move and transform. The water accumulates as edema and swelling of the tissue.

Overconsumption of hot, warm, or dry foods can lead to heat in the stomach and intestines causing constipation, excessive hunger or thirst, and abdominal distention or pain. Patients should avoid overconsumption of alcohol and overeating fatty, greasy, or fried foods, all of which can engender damp heat. Such foods also inhibit the liver qi's coursing and discharge (*shu xie* 疏泄) and causes counterflow which disrupts the spleen's transformative process. The spleen also governs the muscles and flesh, and the muscles and flesh can easily turn to fat if the spleen is out of balance and unable to transform dampness. In that case, the dampness may pour over into the muscles and flesh and stagnate there as added fat. Over-eating foods which cause heat can lead to yang exuberance patterns with symptoms such as high blood pressure, a red face, irritability, and even some types of anxiety. When heat is combined with dampness, it can manifest as gout, weight gain, gallstones, and damp heat skin conditions like shingles, eczema, hives, and psoriasis.

Balanced eating from the biomedical point of view

According to the U.S. Department of Agriculture (USDA)'s 2005 New Food Pyramid Guide, a balanced eating style consists of eating the following foods *in moderation*. (Remember the Chinese doctrine of the mean?) I believe there is ample evidence supporting that this is the basis of healthy eating.

From the point of view of this chart, protein means meat, poultry, seafood, rice, quinoa, legumes: nuts, seeds, and beans.

Whole grains refers to rice, wheat, quinoa, barley, oats, etc.

Dairy refers to milk products of all types. This includes milk, cream, half-and-half, sour cream, clotted cream, yogurt, cheeses of all types, and butter.

The USDA recommends that people eat dairy products primarily to meet the nutritional need for calcium. However, there are many other foods which provide calcium, such as white beans and dark leafy greens. Calcium supple-

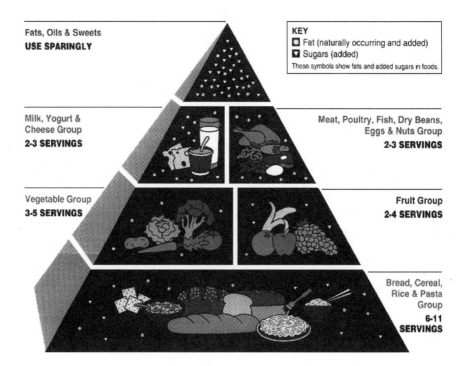

ments are also an alternative for those patients who are lactose intolerant, for those who do eat enough vegetables, or for those who need to avoid eating dairy for any reason. (Also see pages 15-16 for NIH recommendations.)

According to Chinese medicine, milk products are all sweet in flavor (although some are also sour, such as yogurt and some cheeses) and supplement the qi and blood. However, the fattier the milk product, the sweeter the flavor and also the more it engenders fluids. Because milk products are sweet and damping, overconsumption of dairy (or any sweet taste) can damage the moving and transforming function of the spleen leading to the internal accumulation of dampness and phlegm. In my opinion, low-fat dairy may cause less damage to the spleen because it is less sweet and, therefore, less dampening. According to Chinese medicine's temperature classification, cow's milk is neutral. However, chilled cow milk out of the refrigerator is at least cool if not cold. It is also my belief that cow's raised with antibiotics produce milk that is cool. Goat's milk is warm but, like all foods, should nonetheless be consumed in moderation.

Vegetables refer to leafy green vegetables such as kale, collard, chard, mustard and turnip greens, lettuce, and cabbage. They also refer to green beans and peas, root vegetables such as carrots, parsnips, turnips, rutabagas, and potatoes, and gourds and squashes of all kinds.

When eating vegetables, fresh and in season vegetables are preferred. The vegetables one eats should also be varied. One should eat at least five servings of vegetables (and fruit) per day. However, one should avoid overeating raw or juiced vegetables. The ancient Chinese did not can vegetables. They did, however ferment, jar, and store vegetables. Modern research shows the fermentation process, such as that used in the making of sauerkraut and *kim chi*, grows bacteria healthy for the intestines.

Fruits refer to oranges, lemons, grapefruits, and limes, apples, pears, apricots, peaches, and nectarines, melons, such as watermelons, cantaloupe, and cranshaw, pineapple, bananas, etc.

Most fruits are sweet. So avoid overconsumption. It is also better to eat whole fruits instead of juicing. Avoid overconsumption of those raw fruits which are classified in Chinese medicine as cold unless one has a hot stomach and intestines and then only in moderation. Many berries, such as blueberries, are warm.

In Chinese medicine in general, it is common to recommend eating whole, cooked foods, to avoid overeating raw foods, and to avoid juicing as meal replacement. According to Chinese medicine, it is not advisable to overeat raw foods, juices, and dairy products because they are classified as cold and/or dampening.

Before juicers were invented, fruits and vegetables were eaten in their whole form so that most of its fiber was ingested. We would eat the in-season fruit or vegetable freshly picked that day. If we drank the juice, we would do so by holding the piece of fruit over our mouth and squeezing it to allow the cool, sweet juice to flow down our throat. Or we hand squeezed juice, which was laborious, and, therefore, only drank a minimal amount. The advent of juicers has relieved us of this labor, but, if we replace whole food consumption with juice consumption, we reduce the amount of fiber we consume and increase the amount of fruit sugars we consume. Instead of drinking large glasses of juices, advise patients to drink juiced foods in moderation and encourage the patient to eat their five servings of whole vegetables and fruits as often as possible. Serving sizes are one or two pieces of fruit like apples or bananas, one cup of berries, or one to two cups of cooked vegetables.

Practitioners and patient's can use the USDA's 2005 New Food Pyramid Guide to ascertain how many servings of each food group each patient needs. The USDA's website (www.MyPyramid.gov) is easy to navigate, and the new food pyramid is a new model that has been revised to tailor nutritional requirements to individuals needs. This is unlike the old model which was a one-size-fits-all model. This website teaches people in an interactive way to tailor diet choices to their individual nutritional needs. Practitioners should also refer to the appendix in the NIH's free publication number 00-4084, Practical Guide: *Identification, Evaluation and Treatment of Overweight and Obesity in Adults*. The appendix supplies the practitioner with reprintable handouts for patients made for the purpose of guiding them in how to eat a balanced diet and integrate physical activity into daily life.

Understanding carbohydrates, sugars & the glycemic index (GI)

In recent years, low-carbohydrate diets have received a great amount of media attention and have affected the food choices available to consumers. For example, even family and fast food restaurant chains hang signs in their windows advertising low-carbohydrate meals. But instead of providing a healthy diet option, low-carbohydrate Atkins-like meals may actually contribute to weight gain and heart disease due to their extremely high fat content. This is because foods which are high in fat are also high in calories. This segment will address the importance of carbohydrate consumption, how carbohydrate control contributes to weight loss and maintenance, and, conversely, how carbohydrate overconsumption leads to weight gain and other serious health concerns.

How carbohydrates function in the body

Our patients' nonexpert knowledge about carbohydrates varies from person to person. Many know that carbohydrates, found in grains and vegetables, provide energy and that sugars and carbohydrates are somehow related. Lately, common knowledge seems to dictate that carbohydrate indulgence is the main reason for fat storage and weight gain. As a result of this common knowledge, many have cut out carbohydrates altogether not realizing how necessary they are for good health.

Carbohydrates are transformed in the body into an important and essential source of energy necessary for basic cellular and organ function and kinetic muscular activity. Grains are the staple food in a variety of cultures and are the main source of carbohydrates in most diets, along with fruits and vegetables. After consuming a food, the body begins to digest and convert the food into potentially usable energy. Energy which is not used is stored as potential energy. When the body is active, energy fuels activity. During activity, the energy transforms again. If the body is inactive or if the level of activity is disproportionately low compared to the amount of food energy taken in, or the body does not transform that energy, that unused energy is stored. Weight gain occurs as a result of that stored energy going unused.

By classifying the types of food energy sources, practitioners of Chinese medicine recognized long ago what modern nutritionists and diet gurus have recently examined and quantified within the scientific paradigm. We all agree that the types and quantities of energy sources that we consume play an integral part in weight and health maintenance. low-fat diets were born in the 1960s based on the logic that less fat going into the body equals less fat stored in the body. Soon after, Dr. Robert Atkins, MD, asserted that, without receiving a normal supply of carbohydrate energy (while receiving necessary protein and fat), the body would tap into those stored sources of body fat to make up for the shortage. The physiological result of the Atkins and other high protein, low or no carbohydrate diets is that, rather than the body using carbohydrates for energy, it uses fat. However, since the body is designed to use carbohydrates as its main energy source to fuel activity, this diet is prob lematic. High protein and low-fat diets have helped people lose weight, but as it turns out, both of these approaches have unique downfalls which should concern Chinese medical practitioners.

The disadvantages of low-fat & low-carbohydrate diets

Low-fat diets work for weight loss when combined with a healthy exercise routine. Such exercise should consist of at least 30 minutes of cardiovascular exercise at least four times per week in order to burn food energy so that it is not stored as fat. But even for those able to commit to the exercise routine, the weight loss from this low-fat, regular exercise approach comes slowly, and many dieters become frustrated. Part of the frustration results from the limited food choices available for low-fat dieters. The lack of fat in the diet tends to leave dieters feeling hungry shortly after they have eaten a meal. Fats slow down the digestive process, thus allowing the body to use the food energy over an extended period of time and leaving us feeling immediately satiated from the meal and for many hours after. When the dieter feels deprived of certain foods or feels hungry, she or he is more likely to splurge or binge on those forbidden foods which commonly leads to eater guilt and, most frustratingly, negate whatever weight loss had been gained before the splurge. Thus, weight-loss results are further slowed, and the dieter is further frustrated.

Extremely low-carbohydrate diets, like the Atkins' diet which limits daily carbohydrates to fewer than 30 grams per day, result in more dangerous long-term effects but have gained popularity because the eating plan provides immediate and noticeable weight loss results. It appears that Dr. Atkins' claim that drastically limiting carbohydrate intake forces the body to use up stored reserves are true. In fact, this drastic process of ketosis used over a long period of time is well known to humans but is better known by another name: starvation. The intake of protein, fats, and fewer than 30 grams of carbohydrates keeps the body functioning. It also keeps the body from immediately breaking down muscle for usable energy as it normally would under starvation conditions from total food source deprivation (as in anorexics, bulimics, famine victims, unregulated type 1 diabetics, and alcoholics).

Low-carbohydrate dieters like the fast weight loss. However, the cause of the initial weight loss is disputed and deceptive. According to the authors of *The Glucose Revolution*, "The weight you lose is mostly water (that was trapped or held with stored carbohydrates) and eventually muscle as it is broken down to produce glucose [usable energy]. Once you return to your former way of eating [or, in the case of Atkins dieters, once you move from the induction diet to the maintenance diet], you regain a little bit more fat."[13] Regaining lost weight frustrates a dieter, but a cause for more concern is that "the resulting change in body composition to less muscle and more fat

---

[13] Brand-Miller, J., Burani, J., Foster-Powell, K., *The Glucose Revolution Life Plan*, Marlowe & Co. New York, 2001 p. 5.

makes it increasingly difficult to lose weight."[14] So the end result of this eating approach transforms the composition of the body, boosting overall body fat percentage. Bodies with higher percentages of body fat (and, thus, lower percentages of muscle mass) lose weight at a slower pace than bodies with low body fat and high muscle mass ratios. This unhealthy change in ratios is one reason why I caution all of my patients against crash diets and extremely low calorie (under 800 calories/day) diets.

Low-carbohydrate diets allow eaters to consume more of the foods that the USDA, NIH, and low-fat diets caution against. Foods high in fat (and protein), such as cheese, red meat, cream, bacon, and deli meats, keep an eater's belly feeling satisfied and full for longer periods of time. But these dieters often become frustrated with their limited menu options despite the growing number of low-carbohydrate selections.

The *New York Times* has reported that, "The average person eats 50 grams of protein per day, but low-carbohydrate dieters consume 300 grams of protein a day. This increase may raise the risk of heart disease and heart attack by as much as 75 percent,"[15] in part because most high protein foods are also high in fat, especially unhealthy saturated and hydrogenated fats. These unhealthy fats increase low-density lipid (LDL) cholesterol levels leading to atherosclerosis which is a comorbidity factor of overweight and obesity. In addition, people who eat diets higher in fiber found in carbohydrate foods, such as vegetables and whole grains like rice and wheat products, are less likely to get colon cancer. Further, high protein intake can raise acidity levels in the stomach which can lead to acid reflux disease.

The disadvantages of overeating high glycemic index (GI) foods

High GI foods, usually white refined carbohydrate sources, are lower in nutritional quality and have a GI value of greater than 70. Low GI foods have a GI value of lower than 55 and are of higher nutritional quality. High GI foods dump sugars into the blood quickly and overload the body; whereas low GI foods slowly release glucose into the blood and thereby regulate blood sugar and energy levels. The pace at which sugars enter the bloodstream is known as the glycemic load.

The average American eats approximately 138.7 pounds of potatoes per year, 50% of which are consumed fried, and includes 16 pounds of potato

---

[14] *Ibid.*

[15] Brody, Jane E., "The Widening of America, or How Size 4 Became Size 0", *New York Times.* 20 Jan. 2004: 3A.

chips. This is compared to only 23.4 pounds of low GI, dark green, leafy vegetables.[16] When eating a high GI food, such as white potatoes, the blood glucose levels raise quickly and insulin levels rise to make the glucose usable as energy. This provides a burst of energy. In those with diabetes mellitus, these dramatic fluctuations in blood sugar levels and resulting insulin level changes present a serious health concern. Even those who are not diabetic need be concerned with rising and falling glucose levels and insulin production. We have known for some time that obesity can lead to type 2 or so-called adult-onset diabetes, but understanding the way that high GI carbohydrates exhaust the body's production of insulin makes this connection between excess weight, blood sugar level fluctuations, and type 2 diabetes even clearer. In people who are physically active, the energy from high GI foods is quickly burned off and they experience a noticeable decrease in energy as the spiked level of glucose is used up. In people who are inactive, the body will store the energy, leading to weight gain. When blood glucose levels drop so soon after eating, hunger returns. This then leads to overeating which leads to more weight gain.

The advantages of eating low GI foods

The low GI diet is a balanced diet including 25% proteins, 20% healthy fats, and 55% whole carbohydrates derived from grains and vegetables. The glycemic index of a food helps determine how quickly it affects blood sugar levels (which affects energy levels and weight gain) by measuring the quality of the carbohydrate. Eating low GI foods helps regain or maintain dietary balance. Foods with a low GI rating, like long grain rice and spinach, do not cause a marked spike in glucose levels. Instead, the carbohydrate energy is slowly converted to glucose and enters the bloodstream slowly. Because of this slow, steady glucose load, the pancreas' production of insulin is not burned out by a rush of glucose. This even glucose release affects the body in a number of positive ways. The energy gained from foods low on the GI last and is sustained for longer stretches of time. This leaves patients less hungry less often, making them less likely to overeat due to energy overloads and subsequent deprivation (the so-called sugar blues). The addition of protein and/or a healthy fat, like olive oil, to every meal helps slow down the glucose release even more. Therefore, I strongly advise patients to be less concerned about the *quantity* of carbohydrates but more concerned with the *quality* of

---

[16] Putnam, J., Allshouse, J., Kantor L.S., "U.S. Food Supply Trends: More Calories, Refined Carbohydrates and Fat", Winter 2002, p 11 *Food Review* Vol. 25 Issue 3
www.ers.usda.gov/publications/FoodReview/DEC2002/frvol25i3a.pdf accessed 11.24.06

carbohydrates, particularly in terms of their effect on blood sugar and energy levels. Of course, portion control is important for many patients, but eating low GI carbohydrate sources in moderation makes for a more satisfying and balanced meal as opposed to altogether cutting carbohydrates out of the diet.

Other benefits of low GI eating

Interestingly, low GI foods have other health benefits that affect weight control and maintenance, which should be a concern for everyone, not only those with type 1 and 2 diabetes, athletes, or people with weight problems. As noted earlier, eating high GI foods can lead to the unhealthy distribution of fats in the blood and tissue, but low GI foods, in part because they are usually also high in fiber, help to decrease cholesterol levels and naturally decrease the risk of associated health risks like heart disease and diseases of the colon. The more vegetable carbohydrates the patient includes in the diet, the better. This is because most vegetables (except for white potato) have a very low GI. People who eat a low GI lifestyle diet tend to avoid eating processed and fast foods on a regular basis.

Balance is the key to health

Patients should not eliminate carbohydrates from their diet but instead should primarily eat carbohydrates which have a lower GI to achieve a healthy balanced diet. Balance also means well-rounded meals complete with carbohydrates, protein, vegetables, and good fats. Of course, sometimes it is hard to avoid eating high GI foods at weddings, birthdays, or holiday celebrations. When eaten infrequently on occasions like those, high GI foods should be enjoyed!

Eating rice is healthy—in moderation

Rice carbohydrate and GI also deserves more attention. In the old days, rice was hand-hulled and processed leaving much of the bran which is high in healthy oils, protein, and vitamins, especially B vitamins. With the advent of the industrial age, the demand for rice rose substantially. However, the oils in un-milled rice turns rancid. Therefore, manufacturers began removing the bran so that it could be stored longer and shipped further without spoiling. Therefore, the economic value of high quality milled rice has played an important role in its popularity. Rice milling removes most of the above mentioned healthy qualities. However, this rice is often enriched after processing to add back what was lost. Unfortunately, bran is not added back. The missing bran allows for the carbohydrate sugars (of all kinds of grains, wheat included) to pass more quickly into the bloodstream, thus raising blood sugar and body fat levels. In general, rice is an amazingly healthy food. Brown rice and wild rice have a low GI load, while most parboiled rice has a medium load, but highly processed parboiled and all instant rice have a high GI load.

Since the industrial age, people have been eating highly processed, refined grains and wheat (*i.e.*, white bread and white flour) as they have been slowing down their lifestyle by working at desks instead of in the fields. This sedentary lifestyle is prevalent in North America and Europe and even in larger cities in developing countries such as Beijing. It is an interesting fact that China is also facing an obesity epidemic due to poor diet, sedentary lifestyle, and the outdated belief that the more food one eats the richer one is. Ninety million Chinese are obese, and that number is rising steadily. The majority of obesity in China and Japan is found in larger cities where people have desk jobs and cars and eat fast food and milled white rice.

The FDA recommends that people eat at least six ounces of grains per day. Generally, one ounce is one slice of bread, 1/2 cup of cooked rice, pasta, or cooked cereal, or one cup of ready-to-eat/cold cereal. I advise my patients to eat moderate portions of medium GI load rice. A moderate portion size of rice per meal ranges from 1-2 servings (1/2-1 cup cooked) for many people. Very active people may be able to eat more to fuel their increased activity without causing weight gain. For a more complete list of food serving sizes and for more information about serving size appropriateness based upon age, sex, and physical activity level, readers should visit the FDA's new food pyramid website at www.MyPyramid.com.

What Low GI Foods Do For The Body

- Promote and maintain healthy weight loss
- Reduce blood cholesterol levels
- Help reduce the risk of atherosclerosis
- Increase HDL, or good, cholesterol
- Decrease LDL, or bad, cholesterol
- Improve blood sugar control in type 1 and type 2 diabetes
- Increase intake of fiber which results in improved colon health
- Increase intake of greens which contain important folic acid, B vitamins, antioxidants, omega-3 and calcium

Foods That Are Low (<55) On The Glycemic Index

- All meats, fish and nuts

- All vegetables (except white potatoes). Serving size: 1/2 cup cooked. The GI value of most vegetables is negligible so they can be eaten plentifully.

- Long grain basmati rice, converted rice, brown rice, wild rice and long grain parboiled rice. Serving size: 1/2 cup cooked. (Instant rice, puffed rice including rice cakes, arborio and sticky rice have high GI values.)

- Semolina pasta, rice noodles and whole wheat pasta. Serving size: 1/2 cup cooked. These have an even lower GI value than long grain white rice.

- Legumes such as soybeans, chickpeas, lentils, kidney beans, etc. Serving size: 1 cup cooked or dried

- Whole grain breads, pumpernickel, sourdough, stone ground grains, and any bread that does not contain refined white flour. Serving size: 1 slice

- Bulgur, barley, rolled oats, oat bran, granola and muesli. Serving size: 1/2 cup

- Apple, cherries, grapefruit, grapes, kiwi, mango, orange, peach, pear, plum, berries. Serving size: 1 piece, 1/2 cup of juice, 1/2 cup sliced, canned, or cooked with no sugar additives.

- New potatoes, sweet potatoes, taro, and yams rate as moderate (66-69) on the GI when eaten in moderation.

As plated amounts of food vary, so will the GI of any given meal. Therefore, the serving sizes listed above as low GI may not be what actually lands on the plate at a restaurant or at a holiday party. Those servings could be exponentially larger. Thus, I advise patients that in circumstances such as these, they can exercise portion control by making themselves a smaller plate at parties. If at a restaurant or dinner party, one can split the entré with a friend or immediately ask the server to pack half the food to go. This can then be eaten at another meal.

Types of Dieters
& Diet Styles

7

Patients come from a variety of diet style backgrounds and commonly ask questions about the effectiveness and validity of various diet styles. As we counsel patients in a new eating style, it is important to understand how they eat in order to determine what changes should be made. Diet styles vary according to region, culture, education, economics, and political and spiritual belief systems. The following is a summary with commentary describing typical dieters and diet styles commonly encountered in clinical practice.

Types of dieters

Omnivores: These people eat all kinds of food, both plant and animal.
Flexitarians: These people eat mainly vegetarian food but occasionally eat meat or fish.

Chinese medicine classifies the omnivore style as a balanced diet as long as foods are eaten in moderation (especially processed, fatty, greasy, fried and sweets). Omnivore and flexitarian dieters can be very healthy or extremely unhealthy and unbalanced. As with all patients, omnivore and flexitarian food dieters should keep a food diary so we can discern if and how the diet is out of balance. They may need an adjustment of energetic balance of foods in their diet, may need to reduce portion size, or may need to eat more whole grains and to eat at least five servings of varied vegetables daily. Patients should vary food choices and eat fresh, in-season foods as often as possible while avoiding packaged, processed foods, and over-cooked foods.

Atkins dieters: These people eat foods unusually high in protein, especially animal protein, and foods high in saturated fat. They avoid grain-based carbohydrates and eat very little, if any, vegetables or fruit.

Muscle massives: These people eat high protein, low saturated fat foods in order to build muscle mass for weight-training and body-building competitions. Not all muscle massives eat vegetables and fruits regularly.

I find that Atkins dieters and muscle massives tend to exhibit excessive yang conditions due to the unusually high intake of meats (yang) and rich foods (stagnating). Atkins dieters frequently present with damp heat conditions due to overeating high fat foods and meat. They hold weight mainly in the midsection and/or chest. Many have rheumatoid arthritis, gout, gallstones, high blood pressure, and/or high cholesterol. For overall health, many practitioners choose to advise patients against Atkins-type diets, especially for those with high blood pressure and high blood lipid levels because this diet "allows" high fat foods. Patients on these diets tend to weight cycle. This means repeatedly gaining and losing weight, and this is a frustrating experience. So eating more healthfully and losing weight in a moderate, controlled, balanced way is safer and more effective for weight loss maintenance.

Many high protein dieters who drink protein drinks and frequently eat protein bars suffer from hyperacidosis, a.k.a. acid reflux, a stomach condition due to upward counterflow of the stomach qi. In this case, stomach acid flows upward, often burning the esophagus. Happily, this condition is usually easy to treat with acupuncture, Chinese herbs, and diet change. Acupuncture and Chinese herbal treatment should focus on harmonizing the liver and stomach and downbearing counterflow. The practitioner should energetically balance the diet with fish and other yin foods, eliminate protein drinks and meal replacement bars, and advise that the patient avoid overeating protein. The patient should be instructed to eat whole grains and vegetables and to eat at least five servings of varied vegetables and fruits per day.

Junk food junkies: These people eat all processed, frozen, high-fat, high-sodium, greasy, oily fried foods, white, refined flour products, such as white bread, cakes, cookies, and foods high in sugar. The Starchatarian (see below) often fits into this category as well.

This patient needs a complete diet overhaul consisting of many of the suggestions previously discussed in this chapter. Some of these patients will need to take small steps, and some will be able to handle swifter shifts in diet. Practitioners should work with the individual by creating weekly and/or monthly goals for change. Junk food junkies and all patients with a sweet-tooth should be educated about what they can do to beat the sweet cravings.

Start by teaching the patient how sugar affects health and weight. In Western nutrition, the movement of sugar into the bloodstream is described as the glycemic load (GL) dumped into the bloodstream. Keeping the GL low to control blood sugar levels is advisable and is especially important in those with diabetes mellitus, insulin resistance, and metabolic syndrome. Because sugar is transformed into fat, a reduction in GL leads to a reduction in weight gain and helps keep weight off. In Chinese medicine, the weight gain is due to the spleen's inability to transform dampness caused by overconsumption of sugars and sweets. Sugar is classified as cold and dampening in Chinese medicine, and both cold and dampness damage the spleen. When dampness accumulates over time, it congeals into phlegm, and, as we have seen above, excessive fat is nothing other than phlegm dampness in Chinese medicine.

Sugar addiction is a real and important concern. "The American Heart Association's Committee on Nutrition informed health care professionals that sugar consumption promotes obesity and raises triglycerides. Any extra calories are converted into body fat for storage, and sugar is a fuel that delivers calories with great efficiency. Extra fat on the body usually produces extra fat in the blood along with added body weight." Instead, patients should eat regularly throughout the day and avoid large amounts of sugar so that the body will not store so many extra caloires as fat.

Sure, sugar is difficult to give up. We all love and crave the sweets present in many of the products we want to eat. Therefore, I find that it is best to advise patients who consume too much sugar that they

> Acupuncture results in pleasurable brain chemistry without the adverse effects of sugar.

should only reduce their intake rather than go "cold turkey." Sugar stimulates the brain to produce opioid chemicals which in turn stimulates elevated dopamine levels. Patients seek out more sweets as a result of elevated dopamine levels. This urge is the same chemical process that a morphine or heroin addict's brain experiences. Fortunately for sugar addicts, quitting is not nearly as hard. Start to reduce intake by half for a few weeks, then by half again for a week, then in half again. Also support the body with regular acupuncture treatments. Acupuncture has been shown to elevate levels of endomorphin-1, beta endorphin, encephalin, serotonin (the hormone which makes people feel satisfied from eating), and dopamine. In other words, acupuncture results in pleasurable brain chemistry without the adverse effects of sugar.

Patients being only human, will sometimes give in to sweets cravings. So rather then attempting to shame them out of these lapses, practitioners should suggest they satisfy the craving by going to a local bakery, gourmet, or specialty chocolate shop. This way, instead of buying a whole pie or cake, they can buy one slice, or buy just two or three chocolate raspberry truffles instead of buying a whole box of cheap chocolates from the drug store. The result is a potentially lower intake of sugar and caloric intake, and the superior quality chocolate or baked delicacy more substantially satisfies the craving than low quality grocery store or quickie-mart junk food. If your patients try this strategy, they may find as my patients have that they will not need to eat as many sweets or eat them as often.

Another cause for overconsumption of sugar and other junk foods is undereating. Many patients skip breakfast and wait until late in the day to eat lunch or even miss it, blaming a busy day at work. Or they eat lunch at noon and do not eat anything again until 8-9 P.M. When they finally do eat, they gorge on whatever is most convenient. Physiologically, when the patient regularly deprives the body of food and then binges, the body goes into a state-of-emergency and responds by storing calories as fat which is an efficient fuel for later use because it burns slowly. Additionally, glucose is dumped into the blood faster than the body can metabolize it. So it too is turned into stored fat. In my experience, ironically, undereating is a chief cause of being oveweight.

In this case, practitioners should encourage patients to have plenty of healthy foods in the home, at work, and while traveling in order to avoid eating unhealthy junk food snacks or fast food. Another way to feel more satiated is to eat meals slowly. It takes about 20 minutes for the brain to receive the signal of fullness from the stomach. Therefore, patients should be encouraged to eat slowly and mindfully, to savor the flavors of each bite, to smell the aroma, to listen to the sound of the food as they bite into it, and to feel the textures.

Vegetarians: These people eat only plant-derived foods, such as grains, legumes, vegetables, nuts and seeds, and fruits.

Vegans: These people basically eat like a vegetarian but strictly avoid *any* animal and dairy products.

The general public often equates a vegetarian diet with a healthy diet. But just because a patient is a vegetarian does not mean that they eat a healthy, balanced, and varied diet. We must always inquire into exactly what such patients are eating and how their food is prepared. In particular, practitioners should ask patients what their protein sources are. Many times when I ask this question of vegetarians, they respond, "I eat a lot of salad." But my questions cannot end here. I must press further to find out the specific ingredients. If that salad does not have legumes or cheese on it, then it contains little to no protein which every healthy, balanced diet must include in each meal. In this case, we should educate our patients on vegetarian protein sources (nuts, seeds, beans, tofu, tempeh, and some grains such as quinoa and brown rice) and how to integrate them into the diet at every meal. The ingredients in most salads are raw and mostly cold and overeating raw, cold foods damages the spleen. In general, eating no or low protein means these patients are getting no or low yang qi from their food. This underscores the fact that all patients seeking weight loss treatment should keep a food diary so that the practitioner can discern exactly what they are eating and where the diet is out of balance.

In clinical practice, I find that many vegetarians, and especially vegans, suffer from yang and/or blood vacuity. This vacuity is commonly due to the lack of animal protein in the diet. Meat, poultry, and broths made from bones contain strong yang qi and supplement the blood. Furthermore, some vegetarians neglect to eat enough yang protein sources such as legumes and whole grains like rice and quinoa. These patients are often fatigued and overweight from eating too many yin foods and too many processed foods and grains. Yang vacuous patients have pallid skin with dark circles under the eyes, bruise easily, are fatigued, and may more easily sustain broken bones. Because fat is phlegm dampness and phlegm dampness are yin evils, such yang vacuity exacerbates the difficulty of losing weight.

A vegetarian lifestyle is not healthy for all people. If the patient presents a severe qi and blood vacuity, it maybe in the best interest of the patient to advise that she or he begin to eat meat and/or fish. Ask the patient if she or he leads a vegetarian lifestyle for spiritual or health reasons. If the reason is health, ask if the patient would be open to eating small amounts of meat broths and/or small amounts of poultry or fish. If the answer is yes, encourage the slow integration of animal proteins and immediate integration of non-animal sources of qi-supplementing, blood-nourishing foods, such as black beans, orange squashes, leafy green vegetables, and *Gou Qi Zi* (Fructus Lycii).(*Gou Qi Zi* are dried small red berries similar to raisins. In Chinese medicine, *Gou Qi Zi* are both a food and a powerful medicine. In particular, *Gou Qi Zi* are effective for supplementing the blood.) If the patient eats vegetarian for spiritual reasons and, after discussion, is not willing to change their diet, the practitioner must respect that decision. In that case, we can advise other non-animal foods and administer vegetarian herbs to correct the imbalance. However, the patient needs to know that, without eating animal foods, we may not be 100 percent successful.

A fine example of a balanced yang-style, vegetarian-friendly diet is East Indian food. This typically combines rice, chick peas, lentils, and a variety of nuts, all of which are protein sources. Also integral to the distinct flavor of Indian food are warm, aromatic herbs, such cardamom, cinnamon, ginger, cumin, coriander, turmeric, cloves, and chilies. If a vegetarian patient is adventurous, encourage her or him to learn the Indian style of cooking. Any patient with yang vacuity can also drink *masala chai*. *Masala chai* is Indian spiced tea made from cardamom and ginger (and other warming spices depending on the recipe). This should be drunk preferably without milk or one can substitute soy milk or almond milk for cow's milk. The warming, aromatic spices both warm the spleen and help to transform phlegm and dampness. In addition, almonds used for almond milk are sweet but they actually transform dampness and phlegm. Other yang-style, vegetarian-friendly cuisines are Korean, Chinese, and southern Italian. Patients can also experiment with substituting beans, tempeh, and tofu into Mediterranean and North African cuisines.

Ovo-lacto vegetarians: These people eat eggs, dairy products, and vegetarian.

Many ovo-lacto vegetarian patients rely too much on dairy as a protein source. Also, the fats in cheese help them feel satiated. As we have already seen, most forms of dairy are cool and dampening. Therefore, these patients should be counseled to significantly reduce if not eliminate dairy for at least three months and replace the dairy with healthy fats, such as olive oil, to feel satiated. They should also slowly integrate more nuts, seeds, and legumes into their diet for their protein source. Good grain protein sources are quinoa and unrefined rice (a.k.a. brown rice). Ovo-lacto patients should eat protein with every meal and, when eating dairy, should make sure to choose no or low-fat sources. Also, whenever possible, they should choose organic. Chinese medicine classifies goat cheese and goat's milk as warm and, there-fore, not as dampening when eaten in moderation.

Raw foods vegetarians: These people eat only fresh, uncooked vegetables and juices, or vegetables cooked only up to 120 degrees Fahrenheit.

Raw food eaters should be educated to stop eating every food item uncooked. This is because uncooked vegetables tend to be cool or cold and this can be dampening and damaging to the spleen. Rather then eating a diet of entirely raw foods, such patients should primarily eat vegetables which are lightly steamed. They should avoid fruit juices because the excessive dampness in fruit juices impedes the spleen's moving and transforming function, and the glycemic load is too much for the pancreas to metabolize, thus causing weight gain. Some raw foods vegetarians consume an entirely liquid diet. Once these patients begin to eat whole foods again, they will gain weight. So they should be made aware of this fact. However, they should be advised not to be discouraged by this. In my experience, they will eventually stop gaining as long as they eat balanced whole foods and exercise regularly. I suggest that these patients should be encouraged to stay the course because a more balanced eating style will increase health and longevity in the long run.

Macrobiotics: These people eat fresh, cooked vegetarian foods and seaweeds based on yin and yang principles. (However, the specifics of their use of yin and yang varies from Chinese medicine.) Most macrobiotics are mostly vegetarian, although some may eat fish and occasional meat. The foundation and centerpiece of the macrobiotic diet is brown rice. Macrobiotics also eat a number of specifically Japanese foods, such as miso, tamari, certain seaweeds, kanten, nato, and amasake and their food tends to be Japanese in taste. In addition, macrobiotics believe in certain methods of food preparation based on traditional Japanese methods.

Patients who are committed to a macrobiotic style of eating usually eat in a very balanced manner. This style of eating takes considerable time and preparation. If your patient is considering this style of eating, open an encouraging dialogue about what is required to maintain it and inquire if living a proactive macrobiotic lifestyle is a reality for them. If patients cannot devote the time, effort, and planning, make suggestions to help them eat a simpler, healthy diet. For example, by using canned beans instead of always soaking dry beans, they do not have to plan days ahead of time.

Macrobiotics can be a healthy diet for many patients, especially if the person includes some meat, eggs, and fish and is not too doctrinaire about some of the finer points of this lifestyle. Like Chinese medicine, macrobiotics stresses balance and finding one's own yin-yang balance. However, some macrobiotics eat too much salt, and this can be unhealthy over time.

Vegaquarians: These people eat a vegetarian diet that definitely includes fish.

This diet should be balanced like all the others previously discussed. While fish typically contains less fat than most so-called red meats, it can contain too many heavy metals, such as mercury, which are not good for overall health. When eating fish, these patients should be advised to vary the types they eat. Also advise all patients who eat a lot of fish to stay abreast of mercury levels in the fish they choose. One can easily find this information by running a search on the Internet for local or national government mercury level health advisories. These people should also be advised to include other non-animal protein sources in their diets. In addition, for some people, it has become a truth that fish is healthier than meat in any and all instances. However, in Chinese medicine, we believe that overeating any one food or one kind of food can produce imbalance in the body. As I have said before, in Chinese medicine, we believe there are no magic bullets as far as health is concerned, and only eating fish as a source of protein is another form of magic-bullet thinking. Red meat is not bad when eaten in small amounts. It is only overeating red meat that is a problem. So, depending on the patient, the practitioner may want to broach this subject and advise the sparing addition of some lean red meat as well as poultry to the diet.

> In Chinese medicine, we believe that overeating any one food or one kind of food can produce imbalance in the body.

Starchatarians:[17] These people eat a vegetarian diet consisting mainly of bread, potatos, fried foods, and junk vegetarian foods like cookies and cakes. They rarely or never eat vegetables or legumes.

This diet is similar to the junk food junkie's diet, and patients should be advised similarly to avoid overeating starchy, sugary foods. They should include vegetables and protein in every meal.

Encourage all types of vegetarian patients to make sure they eat enough protein and to vary vegetables. Vegetarians often have a hard time eating well when eating out. In this case, they might try eating a little protein at home to avoid overeating and to avoid eating starchatarian style.

Types of diets

The following content is derived from the Federal Citizen Information (FCI) website.[18] The FCI content contains a list of diets types followed by definition and discussion of those types. I have added bracketed commentary.

---

[17] This term was coined by holistic educator and filmmaker Supanova Slom in his DVD entitled *Holistic Wellness for the Hip Hop Generation*, 2003

[18] http://www.pueblo.gsa.gov/cic_text/health/weightloss4life/wtloss.htm, accessed 9.16.06

Fixed-menu diet. A fixed-menu diet provides a list of all the foods the patient will eat. This kind of diet can be easy to follow because the foods are selected for them. But, they provide very few food choices which may make the diet boring and hard to follow away from home. In addition, fixed-menu diets do not teach the food selection skills necessary for keeping weight off. [If patients start with a fixed-menu diet, we should advise that they eventually switch to a plan that helps them learn to make meal choices on their own, such as an exchange-type diet.]

Exchange-type diet. An exchange-type diet is a meal plan with a set number of servings from each of several food groups. Within each group, foods are about equal in calories and can be interchanged. For example, the "starch" category could include one slice of bread or 1/2 cup of oatmeal; each is about equal in nutritional value and calories. If the meal plan calls for two starch choices at breakfast, one could choose to eat two slices of bread, or one slice of bread and 1/2 cup of oatmeal. Exchange-type diet plans have more day-to-day variety and are easier to follow when away from home. The most important advantage is that exchange-type diet plans teach the food selection skills patients need to keep weight off. [This type of diet allows the patient to eat a variety of fresh seasonal foods which is important for energetic balance according to Chinese medicine. The flexibility of this diet is great for those who are vegetarian, kosher, or who have food allergies.]

Prepackaged-meal diet. These diets require the consumer to buy prepackaged meals. Such meals may help them learn appropriate portion sizes. However, they can be costly. Advise the patient that before beginning this type of program they should find out if they need to buy the meals and how much the meals cost. They should also find out whether the program will teach how to select and prepare food, skills that are needed to sustain weight loss. [Aside from portion control, a benefit of these diets is that the foods are prepared reducing shopping and cooking time for busy professionals and commuters. However, many of these frozen or processed foods do not taste very good. Recently, some prepackaged meal plans that can be delivered to your home daily, such as The Zone diet, are fresh and tasty. Unfortunately, many of these types of diets are not vegetarian-friendly or kosher nor are they friendly to those with food allergies. Some patients eat prepackaged frozen diet meals that they buy at the grocery store. Although inexpensive and convenient, many are very high in sodium and low in nutrients. In my clinical experience, patients do not derive quality food qi from this kind of diet; so advise them to eat fresh foods.]

Formula diet. Formula diets or meal replacement diets are weight-loss plans that replace one or more meals with a liquid formula and/or "energy" bar. Most formula diets are balanced diets containing a mix of protein, carbohydrate, and usually a small amount of fat. Formula diets are usually sold as liquid or a powder to be mixed with liquid. Although formula diets are easy to use and do promote short-term weight loss, most people regain the weight as soon as they stop using the formula. In addition, formula diets do not teach how to make healthy food choices, a necessary skill for keeping weight off. [This type of diet lacks quality nutritive qi. Many of these liquid replacement diets contain dairy or soy protein to which some people are allergic. Occasional supplemental use of these liquids or bars can be helpful, especially if the patient needs additional quick energy for working out or playing sports, but, in clinical practice I advise patients to avoid meal replacement diets.]

Questionable diets. Advise the patient to avoid any diet that suggests they eat a certain nutrient, food, or combination of foods to promote easy weight loss. [This includes raw foods diets.] Some of these diets may work in the short term because they are low in calories. However, they are often not well balanced and may cause nutrient [and qi] deficiencies. In addition, they do not teach eating habits that are important for long-term weight management.

Flexible diets. Some programs or books suggest monitoring fat only, calories only, or a combination of the two, with the individual making the choice of both the type and amount of food eaten. This flexible type of approach works well for many people, and teaches how to control what they eat. One drawback of flexible diets is that some do not consider the total diet. For example, programs that monitor fat only often allow people to take in unlimited amounts of excess calories from sugars, and therefore do not lead to weight loss. [The lack of consideration for total diet contributes to an unbalanced diet. If the patient consumes excess sugar, the diet will lead to phlegm dampness in the body.]

It is important to advise patients to choose an eating plan they can live with. The plan should teach them how to select and prepare healthy foods, as well as how to maintain their new weight. Remember that many people tend to regain lost weight. Eating a healthful and nutritious diet combined with regular physical activity, helps to prevent weight regain.

Diet style change is lifestyle change

Adopting a different eating style is actually a change in lifestyle for our patients, and this usually requires us practitioners to consistently and encouragingly coach them. When I counsel my patients about change, I support their effort to change by saying: "You are transforming your qi and your life. The transformative process takes patience, perseverance, and compassion. So, as you embark on a new way of eating (or any new habit), be kind to yourself if you slip into an old habit. Just acknowledge the awareness that you slipped and explore why. Do not beat yourself up. Instead, ask yourself questions like: Was it because I had no food in the house that I went to a fast food restaurant? If so, how can I plan to stock my refrigerator and cabinets to avoid eating fast foods? Was I feeling emotionally vulnerable when I ate that entire box of cookies? What healthier choice can I make to feel better when I am emotionally vulnerable? Then, after you have acknowledged your awareness, learned why you made the mistake, and prepare yourself how to do better next time, inhale and exhale to let go of the mistake. Keep in mind that each new moment offers the opportunity to 'begin again.'[19]

[19] The "begin again" term was coined by one of my favorite mindfulness meditation teachers, Sharon Salzberg.

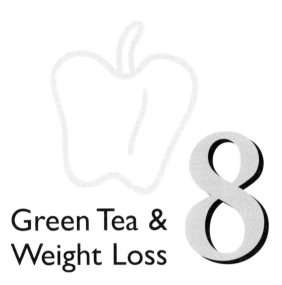

Green Tea & Weight Loss

8

One could hardly write a book about Chinese medicine and weight loss and not include a chapter on green tea. This is because A) green tea is the dominant tea drunk in China. In fact, green tea drinking is so ubiquitous in China, it is hard to walk into any room without finding at least one thermos bottle of hot green tea. And B) there has been so much promotion of green tea for weight loss in the media in recent years.

Green tea refers to the the beverage made from the steeped unfermented leaves of the plant *Camellia sinensis*. According to one Chinese legend, this plant was brought from India to China by the originator of Ch'an or Zen Buddhism, Bodhidharma. However, this legend may only refer to the drinking of tea for staying awake (as through long periods of nocturnal meditation). Historians believe the earliest records of tea-drinking in the world are found in China, with recorded tea use there dating back to the the first millennium BCE. During the Han dynasty (206 BCE-220 CE), tea was being used as medicine, while the use of tea as a beverage drunk for pleasure on social occasions dates from the Tang dynasty (618-907) or earlier.[20]

According to modern research, regularly drinking green tea can:

- Lower cholesterol
- Increase thermogenesis (the body's rate of burning calories)
- Enhance fat oxidation

[20] "History of Tea in China" http://en.wikipedia.org/wiki/History_of_tea_in_China accessed 1.25.07

Green tea contains high concentrations of catechins. Catechins are poly-phenolic antioxidant plant metabolites, specifically flavonoids called flavan-3-ols. These compounds work with other chemicals to intensify levels of fat oxidation and thermogenesis where heat is created in the body by burning fuels such as fat. Green tea also causes carbohydrates to be released slowly, preventing sharp increases in blood insulin levels. It is also thought that the catechins in green tea help prevent obesity by inhibiting the movement of glucose into fat cells. Epigallocatechin gallate (EGCG) is thought to be one of the especially active weight loss, antiadiposity components in green tea.[21] These claims have been substantiated by both animal and human studies.

Animal studies

The University of Chicago's Tang Center for Herbal Medical Research on epigallocatechins (EGCG) showed that blood levels of glucose, lipids, and cholesterol were reduced and that fat deposits under the skin of the abdomen were also reduced. Another green tea weight-loss study described in the health section of the MSN Website also found that green tea extract improved the metabolism of glucose and lipids which is beneficial for weight loss. And further, there have been a number of green tea weight-loss studies in animal models done on the ability of green tea extract to lower blood sugar.[22] In one particular study, conducted by Abdul Dulloo from the Institute of Physiology at the University of Fribourg in Switzerland, researchers exposed a particular type of fatty tissue from rats to caffeine and to green tea extract containing small concentrations of caffeine. Green tea containing caffeine significantly increased thermogenesis by 28-77 percent depending on dose, whereas caffeine alone resulted in no significant increase.[23]

Human studies

In one green tea weight-loss study in humans, oolong tea or green tea extract resulted in an average increase in energy used by the body of 3-4 percent. According to the Linus Pauling Institute, this effect of green tea weight loss is "apparently due to increased fat oxidation and thermogenesis."

---

[21] "Green Tea and Weight Loss" http://www.japanesegreenteaonline.com/weightloss.htm accessed 1.26.07
[22] "Green Tea Weight Loss – Backed by Science?" http://www.vitaminstohealth.com/green-tea-weight-loss.html accessed 1.26.07
[23] "Drinking Green Tea May Help You Lose Weight"
http://www.webmd.com/contents/article/22/1728_55919.htm?z=1671_00000_5022_pe_01 accessed 1.26.07

Thermogenesis refers to energy used in heat production that is not related to resting metabolism or physical activity. In another study, different groups of people were given caffeine to see how that compared to green tea in thermogenesis. The people taking the green tea had higher thermogenesis than those taking the equivalent amount of caffeine without green tea catechins.[24] In this same study, the researchers indicated that their findings have substantial implications for weight control. A four percent overall increase in 24-hour energy expenditure was attributed to the green tea extract. However, the research found that this extra expenditure took place during the daytime. This led them to conclude that, since thermogenesis contributes 8-10 percent of daily energy expenditure in a typical subject, that this four perecent overall increase in energy expenditure due to the green tea actually translated to a 35-43 percent increase in daytime thermogenesis.[25]

One of the most recent human studies on green tea and weight loss was published in the January 2005 issue of the *American Journal of Clinical Nutrition.* In this study, researchers looked at the effects of catechins on body fat reduction and weight loss in a group of 35 Japanese men. The men had similar weights based on their BMI and waist sizes. The men were divided into two groups. For three months, the first group drank a bottle of oolong tea fortified with green tea extract containing 690 milligrams of catechins, and the other group drank a bottle of oolong tea with 22 milligrams of catechins. During this time, the men ate identical breakfasts and dinners and were instructed to control their calorie and fat intake at all times. Therefore, the overall total diets

> Catechins in green tea not only help burn calories and lower LDL cholesterol but may also be able to mildly reduce body fat.

were similar. After three months, the study showed that the men who drank the green tea extract lost more weight (a mean loss of 5.3 pounds vs. 2.9 pounds) and experienced a significantly greater decrease in BMI, waist size, and total body fat. In addition, LDL cholesterol went down in the men who drank the green tea extract. The researchers said that these results indicate that catechins in green tea not only help burn calories and lower LDL cholesterol but may also be able to mildly reduce body fat. According to Tomonori Nagao *et al.* of the Health Care Products Research Laboratories in Tokyo, "These results suggest that catechins contribute to the prevention of and improvement in various lifestyle-related diseases, particularly obesity."[26]

---

[24] "Green Tea and Weight Loss, *op. cit.*
[25] "Green Tea Extract Increases Metabolism" http://thyroid.about.com/cs/dietweightloss/a/greentea.htm accessed 1.26.07
[26] "Green Tea Fights Fat" http://onhealth.webmd.com/script/main/art.asp?articlekey=55970 accessed 1.26.07

To date, there have been no studies done on long-term green tea weight loss, and, like any product that has a beneficial effect, there is no use using it and then living on junk food. That would counteract some, if not all, of green tea's weight-loss benefits. Nevertheless, I believe that regularly drinking green tea and/or taking a dietary supplement containing green tea extract can help in losing weight.

In order to incorporate the benefits of green tea into a weight-loss regime, one can simply drink one cup of tea with each meal. Tea by itself only has four calories per serving, and it is most healthy when consumed with nothing added. The two types of tea which have received the most research in China and Japan regarding weight loss are Pu-erh and Oolong[27], but all types of tea offer a low-calorie alternative to commercial beverages.

[27] "Health Benefits: Green Tea" http://www.generationtea.com/health.htm accessed 1.26.07

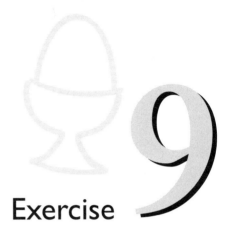

Exercise

Chinese medicine has long recommended regular physical activity as a way to cultivate and maintain wellness. As the famous Chinese doctor and longevity specialist Ge Hong said almost 1,700 years ago: "The [leather] hinges of a moving door never rots, and flowing water never stagnates." As another example of the Chinese people's early understanding of the important of exercise, 25 years or so ago, exercise manuals were unearthed in China along with a cache of medical books from a 2,500 year-old tomb. However, in premodern China, most people were agriculturists who worked in the fields, and most Chinese had only one mode of transportation — their feet. Even getting water for cooking, drinking, and washing required going to the well, stream, or river and carrying it back home in buckets. Similarly, fuel had to be collected and sometimes chopped or cut. As a result of this abundance of physical activity, there was little need for practitioners of Chinese medicine to create a specific system of weight-loss exercise. (For the upper classes and those sequestered in monasteries, there were martial arts, qigong, and tai chi to keep them healthy and fit.) However, today few of us get routine physical exercise just by going about our daily activities. Instead, most of us have to find and engage in some sort of planned physical exercise.

> Today few of us get routine physical exercise just by going about our daily activities. Instead, most of us have to find and engage in some sort of planned physical exercise.

Unfortunately, only 26 percent of U.S. adults engage in vigorous leisure-time physical activity three or more times per week (defined as periods of vigorous physical activity lasting 10 minutes or more). About 59 percent of adults do *no* vigorous physical activity at all in their leisure time.[28] Happily, there is no lack of contemporary research and experience that we can use to help tutor our modern patients on the role of exercise in healthy, sustained weight loss.

The Center for Disease Control (CDC) states that, "Regular physical activity and physical fitness contribute toward health, well-being, and maintenance of a healthy body weight." Physical activity is defined by the CDC as "any bodily movement produced by skeletal muscles resulting in energy expenditure,"[29] and they define physical fitness as "a set of attributes a person has in regards to a person's ability to perform physical activities that require aerobic fitness, endurance, strength, or flexibility and is determined by a combination of regular activity and genetically inherited ability."[30] More energy expenditure results from engaging in fitness activities (like aerobics, biking, soccer) than from everyday physical activity (like walking the dog or climbing stairs).

Energy expenditure is measured in terms of calories. One thousand calories equals one kilocalorie, and a kilocalorie is defined as the amount of heat necessary to raise one gram of water one degree centigrade. When we see "calories" on a food label, it actually means kilocalories. According to the CDC, 3,500 kilocalories of food energy equal one pound of body weight.[31]

In physics, the first law of thermodynamics states that energy is neither created nor destroyed; it simply changes form/transforms. Kilocalories are a form of energy which must be used or burned by the body or it is stored in a transformed state as adipose tissue. This adipose tissue is potential energy which intrinsically possesses the potential for transformation. Substantial amounts of heat from kinetic energy (usually derived through physical activity) transforms adipose tissue resulting in weight loss.

The 2005 *USDA Guidelines for Americans* show that, "A sedentary lifestyle increases risk for overweight and obesity and many chronic diseases, including coronary artery disease, hypertension, type 2 diabetes, osteoporosis, and certain types of cancer. Overall, mortality rates from all causes of death are

---

[28] http://win.niddk.nih.gov/statistics/index.htm#other accessed 1.25.07
[29] http://www.cdc.gov/nccdphp/dnpa/physical/terms/index.htm accessed 10.18.06
[30] *Ibid.*
[31] *Ibid.*

lower in physically active people than in sedentary people. Also, physical activity can aid in managing mild to moderate depression and anxiety."[32]

Counseling our patients on the benefits & necessity of regular physical exercise

In counseling my patients on the benefits and necessity of regular physical exercise, I typically rely heavily on the following NIH and AHA recommendations.

NIH Guidelines

Physical activity should be an integral part of weight loss therapy and weight maintenance. Initially, moderate levels of physical activity for 30-45 minutes 3-5 days per week should be encouraged.

Most weight loss occurs because of decreased caloric intake. Sustained physical activity is most helpful in the prevention of weight regain. In addition, physical activity is beneficial for reducing risks for cardiovascular disease and type 2 diabetes, beyond that produced by weight reduction alone.

Many people live sedentary lives, have little training or skills in physical activity, and are difficult to motivate toward increasing their activity. For these reasons, starting a physical activity regimen may require supervision for some people. The need to avoid injury during physical activity is a high priority. Extremely obese persons may need to start with simple exercises that can be intensified gradually. The practitioner must decide whether exercise testing for cardiopulmonary disease is needed before embarking on a new physical activity regimen. This decision should be based on a patient's age, symptoms, and concomitant risk factors.

For most obese patients, physical activity should be initiated slowly, and the intensity should be increased gradually. Initial activities may be increasing small tasks of daily living such as taking the stairs or walking or swimming at a slow pace. With time, depending on progress, the amount of weight lost, and functional capacity, the patient may engage in more strenuous activities. Some of these include fitness walking, cycling, rowing, crosscountry skiing, aerobic dancing, and jumping rope.

Jogging provides a high-intensity aerobic exercise, but it can lead to orthopedic injury. If jogging is desired, the patient's ability to do this must

[32]USDA *Guidelines for Americans*, 2005 Chapter 4
http://www.health.gov/dietaryguidelines/dga2005/document/html/chapter4.htm accessed 10.19.06

first be assessed. The availability of a safe environment for the jogger is also a necessity. Competitive sports, such as tennis and volleyball, can provide an enjoyable form of physical activity for many, but again, care must be taken to avoid injury, especially in older people . . . a moderate amount of physical activity can be achieved in a variety of ways.

People can select activities that they enjoy and that fit into their daily lives. Because amounts of activity are functions of duration, intensity, and frequency, the same amounts of activity can be obtained in longer sessions of moderately intense activities (such as brisk walking) as in shorter sessions of more strenuous activities (such as running). A regimen of daily walking is an attractive form of physical activity for many people, particularly those who are overweight or obese. The patient can start by walking 10 minutes three days a week and can build to 30-45 minutes of more intense walking at least three days a week and increase to most, if not all, days. With this regimen, an additional 100-200 kilocalories per day of physical activity can be expended. Caloric expenditure will vary depending on the individual's body weight and the intensity of the activity. This regimen can be adapted to other forms of physical activity, but walking is particularly attractive because of its safety and accessibility. With time, a larger weekly volume of physical activity can be performed that would normally cause a greater weight loss if it were not compensated by a higher caloric intake.

Reducing sedentary time, i.e., time spent watching television or playing video games, is another approach to increasing activity. Patients should be encouraged to build physical activities into each day. Examples include leaving public transportation one stop before the usual one, parking farther than usual from work or shopping, and walking up stairs instead of taking elevators or escalators. New forms of physical activity should be suggested, such as gardening, walking a dog daily, or new athletic activities. Engaging in physical activity can be facilitated by identifying a safe area to perform the activity (such as community parks, gyms, pools, and health clubs). However, when these sites are not available, an area of the home can be identified and perhaps outfitted with equipment such as a stationary bicycle or a treadmill. Health care professionals should encourage patients to plan and schedule physical activity one week in advance, budget the time necessary to do it, and document their physical activity by keeping a diary and recording the duration and intensity of exercise.

The following are examples of activities at different levels of intensity:

- A moderate amount of physical activity is roughly equivalent to physical activity that uses approximately 150 calories of energy per day, or 1,000 calories per week.

- For the beginner, or someone who leads a very sedentary lifestyle, very light activity would include increased standing activities, room painting, pushing a wheelchair, yard work, ironing, cooking, and playing a musical instrument.

- Light activity would include slow walking (24 min./mile), garage work, carpentry, house cleaning, child care, golf, sailing, and recreational table tennis.

- Moderate activity would include walking a 15-minute mile, weeding and hoeing a garden, carrying a load, cycling, skiing, tennis, and dancing.

- High activity would include jogging a mile in 10 minutes, walking with a load uphill, tree felling, heavy manual digging, basketball, climbing, and soccer.

- Other key activities would include flexibility exercises to attain full range of joint motion, strength or resistance exercises, and aerobic conditioning.[33]

American Heart Association Guidelines For Cardiovascular Exercise

Cardiovascular exercise defined

- The American Heart Association recommends cardiovascular exercise four times a week for 40 minutes per time nonstop. If that does not help the patient lose weight, adjust by exercising more days, or for longer periods of time and in patients who are able, increase intensity.

Target heart rates (HR)

- To receive the benefits of physical activity, it is important not to tire too quickly. Pacing yourself is especially important if you have been inactive.

- Target heart rates let you measure your initial fitness level and monitor your progress in a fitness program. This approach requires measuring your pulse periodically as you exercise and staying within 50-75 percent of your maximum heart rate. This range is called your target heart rate.

continued

---

[33] NIH Practical Guide: *Identification, Evaluation and Treatment of Overweight and Obesity in Adults*, p. 28-30

American Heart Association Guidelines For Cardiovascular Exercise (*cont.*)

What is an alternative to target heart rates?

- Some people cannot measure their pulse or do not want to take their pulse when exercising. If this is true for you, try using a "conversational pace" to monitor your efforts during moderate activities like walking. If you can talk and walk at the same time, you are not working too hard. If you can sing and maintain your level of effort, you are probably not working hard enough. If you get out of breath quickly, you are probably working too hard, especially if you have to stop and catch your breath.

When should I use the target heart rate?

- If you participate in more vigorous activities like brisk walking and jogging, the "conversational pace" approach may not work. Then try using the target heart rate. It works for many people, and it is a good way for health professionals to monitor your progress.

The table below shows estimated target heart rates for different ages. Look for the age category closest to yours, then read across to find your target heart rate.

Age	Target HR Zone 50-75%	Average Maximum Heart Rate 100%
20 years	100-150 beats per minute	200 beats per minute
25 years	98-146 beats per minute	195 beats per minute
30 years	95-142 beats per minute	190 beats per minute
35 years	93-138 beats per minute	185 beats per minute
40 years	90-135 beats per minute	180 beats per minute
45 years	88-131 beats per minute	175 beats per minute
50 years	85-127 beats per minute	170 beats per minute
55 years	83-123 beats per minute	165 beats per minute
60 years	80-120 beats per minute	160 beats per minute
65 years	78-116 beats per minute	155 beats per minute
70 years	75-113 beats per minute	150 beats per minute

Your maximum heart rate is approximately 220 beats per minute minus your age. The figures above are averages. Therefore, they should be used only as general guidelines.

Note: A few high blood pressure medications lower the maximum heart rate and thus the target zone rate. If you are taking such medicine, call your physician to find out if you need to use a lower target heart rate.

How should I pace myself?

When starting an exercise program, aim at the lowest part of your target zone (50 percent) during the first few weeks. Gradually build up to the higher part of your target zone (75 percent). After six months or more of regular exercise, you may be able to exercise comfortably at up to 85 percent of your maximum heart rate. However, you do not have to exercise that hard to stay in shape.[34]

Target Heart Rates reproduced with permission of www.americanheart.org

Frequently asked questions my patients ask me about exercise

Q: I am going to yoga (or tai chi, qigong) classes but not losing weight. Why?

A: Yoga, tai chi, and qigong are excellent for stretching, strengthening, and toning as well as cultivating qi. However, many styles of yoga (tai chi, qigong) are not cardiovascular exercise. Check your heart rate about 30 minutes into the class to figure out if you are getting a cardiovascular work-out. If you are not getting a cardiovascular work-out, it is still beneficial in many ways to stick with yoga. In that case, just add some sort of regular cardiovascular exercise to your work-out schedule.

Q: Is it more effective to weight train first or do cardiovascular exercise first?

A: Do cardiovascular exercise first before strength training to burn calories more effectively during strength training. If you wait to use weights, you will not fatigue your muscles by doing strength training first, and this may hinder the amount of time and energy you need to dedicate towards cardiovascular exercise.

Q: How can I flatten and strengthen my abdominal muscles?

A: Do abdominal exercises immediately after cardiovascular exercise to maximize calorie burning potential. Always remember to exhale as you do any

---

[34] www.americanheart.org *Target Heart Rates* http://www.americanheart.org/presenter.jhtml?identifier=4736 accessed 5.10.06

abdominal crunches. Also take care not to strain your neck. Place your fingertips, not the whole hand, behind the head and maintain a light fingertip touch during the crunch. Imagine that you are lifting yourself from your torso, not your head. Full sit-ups can cause serious injury to the neck and low back. Crunches are safer and effective. Abdominal muscles attach to support the low back and, when strong, can help eliminate or manage low back pain. Diet has more to do with abdominal weight loss or gain then most other factors. So make sure to eat a healthy, balanced diet and avoid junk food.

Q: I have chronic pain. So how can I exercise?

A: Start by walking five minutes a day. Even if you walk inside the home, it slowly builds energy and strength. Consult with an exercise expert, physical therapist, or fitness trainer to help design an exercise routine to fit your needs. Be careful not to overdo it and cause more pain which can lead to a set-back. Take it one step at a time. Also, get acupuncture to ease the pain. It works.

Q: How can I avoid exercise-induced injury?

A: Always stretch before and after you work out. Warm up with at least 10 minutes of cardiovascular exercise before using weights. Take it slow and easy for at least the first few weeks. You can build up strength and endurance over time. The quality of the work-out is more important then the quantity of weight or repetitions. If you become injured, first rest the area for at least a few days and get acupuncture for the pain. Then, when you are healed, hire a personal trainer for a few sessions. Discuss your fitness goals and the injuries and let them teach you the proper body mechanics for exercise. Then you can go back to exercising on your own. Spending the money on an instructor may save you in physician and acupuncture bills, not to mention saving you from pain which can also disrupt your work-out schedule.

Weight Loss Case Studies 10

The following case studies are taken from my clinic files. Obviously, I have had to change some information in order to protect my patients' privacy. Readers should note that I only use ready-made Chinese herbal medicines in my practice.

Case #1

The patient was a 38 year-old single, professional female with no children. Her height was 5′ 5″ and she weighed 165, with a BMI of 27. Her chief complaint was "fluid imbalance." I treated her for two months with acupuncture once per week, and then we adjusted the treatment schedule to once every two weeks. This regimen was combined with Chinese herbs and Chinese dietary therapy. She took the Chinese herbs in ready-made form three times per day, and I changed the herbal formula according to the changes in her energy over the course of treatment. I also made dietary adjustments on an *ad hoc* basis. The patient lost 10 pounds in two months and continues to lose weight.

Signs & symptoms: The patient's lower legs, ankles, and hands were extremely swollen. The patient was fatigued, had cold hands and feet, bruised easily, and was extremely irritable. In addition, she said she had zero libido and a poor appetite. During menstruation, she had bleeding gums when she brushed her teeth, lower abdominal cramps, clots in her menstruate, low back soreness, and breast distention. She also said she was depressed during her menstrual period. The patient woke nightly to urinate. She also had jaw tightness and night-time bruxism.

Tongue: Dusky pale, swollen and enlarged with teeth-marks on its edges, and thick, white fur

Pulse: Deep, fine, and bowstring

Pattern discrimination: Spleen-kidney yang vacuity with qi stagnation, blood stasis, and food stagnation

Analysis of signs & symptoms: The fatigue, cold hands and feet, easy bruising, bleeding gums during menstruation, swollen tongue, fine pulse, and generalized edema all indicate spleen qi vacuity. The low back soreness, nocturia, and lack of libido plus the deep pulse all indicate kidney yang vacuity. The irritability, depression, breast distention, tight jaw, bruxism, dysmenorrheal, and bowstring pulse all indicate liver depression qi stagnation. The clots in the menstruate suggest an element of blood stasis, while the thick, white tongue fur and poor appetite suggest food stagnation.

Treatment principles: Fortify the spleen and supplement the qi, supplement the kidneys and invigorate yang, course the liver and resolve depression, quicken the blood and abduct food

On the first visit, I asked the woman to begin keeping a food diary. This showed that she consumed several servings of dairy products daily. She also ate a significant amount of raw foods and white flour products. I advised that she stop consuming dairy products for two months and eat only whole grain wheat products in moderation. The patient agreed to follow my instructions. After only two weeks of this diet, she lost three pounds. The swelling in her hands completely abated within the same timespan, while the swelling in the legs and ankles reduced.

Acupuncture: Although points varied from treatment to treatment depending on the patient's main complaints at the time of treatment, the basic treatment consisted of:

Zu San Li (St 36) and *Pi Shu* (Bl 20) to fortify the spleen and
   supplement the qi
San Yin Jiao (Sp 6) and *Shen Shu* (Bl 23) with moxibustion to
   supplement the kidneys and invigorate yang
Tai Chong (Liv 3) and *He Gu* (LI 4) to course the liver and rectify the qi
Zhong Wan (CV 12) and *Liang Men* (St 21) to abduct food and
   disperse stagnation

Further, the combination of *San Yin Jiao* and *He Gu* quickens the blood and dispels stasis.

Chinese medicinals: *Bu Zhong Yi Qi Wan* (Supplement the Center & Boost the Qi Pills), *Shen Qi Wan* (Kidney Qi Pills), and Black Dragon (a ready-made medicine available from Blue Poppy Herbs)

The ingredients of *Bu Zhong Yi Qi Wan* fortify the spleen and boost the qi. However, this formula also harmonizes the liver and spleen and rectifies and frees the flow of the qi mechanism in general. *Shen Qi Wan* supplements the kidneys and invigorates yang. However, it contains medicinals to fortify the spleen, quicken the blood, and seep dampness. Black Dragon contains ingredients which fortify the spleen and supplement the qi, harmonize the liver and rectify the qi, abduct food and disperse stagnation, and quicken the blood and dispel stasis.

Case #2

The patient was a married, professional female aged 32 with no children. She was 5′ 7″ and weighed 160 pounds, with a BMI of 25 on her first visit. This woman's goal was to lose 20 pounds. She commuted three hours every day to and from work and worked long hours which prohibited her from regularly cooking and eating food at home as well as from a regular exercise routine. Consequently, the patient ate out very often. Her work schedule also interfered with regular acupuncture appointments. Nevertheless, this woman lost five pounds in the first five weeks of treatment, during which time she received five acupuncture treatments, took Chinese herbs, and changed her diet the best she could based on our counseling sessions. However, soon thereafter, this woman's weight fluctuated up and down by a few pounds because she could not stay consistent with acupuncture, herbs, diet, or exercise due to her work lifestyle. She was also on birth control pills which is known to cause weight gain and prevent weight loss. About six weeks into treatment, she decided to go off the birth control for weight loss and because she and her husband wanted to have a child within the next year. Even though our success was low in terms of weight loss, I have chosen to present this patient so that the reader can compare results with other cases who received consistent treatment and more thoroughly adopted the lifestyle changes I recommended.

Signs & symptoms: The patient was unable to lose weight, craved sweets, and had a history of acid reflux for which she was taking prescription medication daily. She had persistent heartburn and flatulence which worsened when she was premenstrual. She also had a history of chronic sinus congestion for which she had surgery. However, the surgery had only resulted in minor relief. The patient reported feeling irritable and had frequent cold sores on her lips. She also had chronic muscular tension in the back of her neck and shoulders.

Tongue: Pale with slightly red tip and swollen

Pulse: Deep, bowstring, and forceless

Pattern discrimination: Liver-spleen disharmony with depressive heat in the stomach and lungs and phlegm dampness

Analysis of signs & symptoms: The craving for sweets, pale, swollen tongue, and forceless pulse all indicate spleen qi vacuity, while the PMS, chronic muscular tension, and bowstring pulse all indicate liver depression qi stagnation. The red-tipped tongue, sinus congestion, heartburn, and acid reflux all indicate depressive heat floating upward. The fact that the woman was overweight and her pulse was, therefore, deep, was enough to posit the presence of phlegm dampness.

Treatment principles: Harmonize the liver, spleen, and stomach, clear heat, transform phlegm, and eliminate dampness

Acupuncture:

> *Tai Chong* (Liv 3) and *He Gu* (LI 4) to course the liver and rectify the qi
> *Tai Bai* (Sp 3) and *Zu San Li* (St 36) to fortify the spleen and supplement the qi
> *Tian Shu* (St 25), *Zhong Wan* (CV 12), and *Qu Chi* (LI 11) to clear heat from the yang ming
> *Dan Zhong* (CV 17) and *Jian Jing* (GB 21) to downbear counterflow to treat both the heartburn and neck and shoulder tension
> *Feng Long* (St 40) and *Zhong Wan* to transform phlegm and eliminate dampness

Chinese medicinals: *Xiao Chai Hu Tang Wan* (Minor Bupleurum Decoction Pills), *Xiao Yao Wan* (Rambling Pills), and Black Dragon®.

> *Xiao Chai Hu Tang Wan* harmonizes the liver, spleen, and stomach, clears heat from the liver, stomach, and lungs, transforms phlegm and eliminates dampness

Xiao Yao Wan harmonizes the liver and spleen, transforms and seeps
  dampness
Black Dragon® supplements the spleen, rectifies the qi, and harmonizes
  and clears the stomach

In addition, I advised the patient to cook at home as much as possible and
bring home-cooked food to work. I also asked her to eliminate raw foods from
her diet for three whole months. After that, I said she could eat raw foods in moderation. I also told her to eat whole grains in moderation and eliminate refined
flour and sugar. To clear heat, I suggested that she reduce her consumption of
both hot, spicy and oily, fatty foods. Further, I recommended that the woman
increase her physical activity and exercise as much as possible, for instance, taking
the stairs instead of the elevator, parking farther away from store entrances, etc.

Case #3

This patient was a 45 year-old, white-collar professional who lived with her
life partner. She was 5′ 8″ and weighed 162 pounds, with a BMI of 25. I was
already treating this patient for other health issues, many of which had been
resolved, when she asked me to assist her weight loss. The woman was
already eating well and exercising several times per week with a personal
trainer. However, she was not losing much weight. Working with me, the
patient lost five pounds in one month by taking Chinese herbs combined
with diet and exercise. She said that the herbs gave her more energy to opti-
mize her workouts and she felt less stressed. She only had one acupuncture
treatment over that month. She continued taking Chinese herbs and, within
another month, lost another five pounds.

Signs & symptoms: This woman's main symptoms were fatigue, irritability,
minor depression, low libido, and weak, achy knees.

Tongue: Dusky pale, fat and enlarged with teeth-marks on its edges, and
white fur

Pulse: Fine, forceless, and bowstring

Pattern discrimination: Spleen-kidney yang vacuity with liver depression qi
stagnation and phlegm dampness

Analysis of signs & symptoms: As stated above, being overweight itself indicates
phlegm dampness in Chinese medicine. Fatigue is the hallmark symptom of qi

vacuity, and the spleen is the source of engenderment and transformation of the qi. This is confirmed by the swollen, enlarged tongue, and the fine, forceless pulse. The irritability, depression, and bowstring pulse indicate liver depression qi stagnation, and the low libido coupled with the woman's age and sore, achy knees indicate kidney yang vacuity.

Treatment principles: Fortify the spleen and boost the qi, supplement the kidneys and warm yang, course the liver and rectify the qi, transform phlegm and eliminate dampness

Acupuncture:

> *Tai Chong* (Liv 3) and *He Gu* (Li 4) to course the liver and rectify the qi
> *Zu San Li* (St 36) and *Zhong Wan* (CV 12) to fortify the spleen and
>   supplement the qi
> *Feng Long* (St 40) and *Zhong Wan* to transform phlegm and eliminate
>   dampness
> *Fu Liu* (Ki 7) and *Shen Shu* (Bl 23) with moxibustion to supplement the
>   kidneys and warm yang
> *Yin Tang* (M-HN-3) was added to help quiet the spirit and reduce stress.

Chinese medicinals: *Liu Jun Zi Wan* (Six Gentlemen Pills), *Shen Qi Wan* (Kidney Qi Pills), and Black Dragon®

> *Liu Jun Zi Wan* fortifies the spleen and supplements the qi, transforms
>   phlegm and eliminates dampness
> *Shen Qi Wan* supplements the kidneys and warms yang
> Black Dragon® harmonizes the liver, supplements the spleen, and strong-
>   ly frees the flow of the qi mechanism

In addition, I recommended that this patient continue her healthy, balanced diet and continue her exercise routine, with a focus on cardiovascular exercise. I also suggested that she reduce stress by taking breaks at work and taking more time off.

Case #4

This patient was a 33 year-old female who resided with her partner. She originally came to me because she had had a series of miscarriages. In addition, the woman had been trying to lose weight for many months. This weight loss was slow but steady. I treated the patient for her reproductive problems, but, she noticed that her weight had dropped two times as fast during or after getting acupuncture, taking Chinese herbs, and eating a diet based on her pattern discrimination. When she came to me she was 5' 5" and weighed 160 pounds, with a BMI of 27. Within five weeks of treatment, the patient lost 10 pounds and continues to safely lose weight. We will stop her weight loses when she reaches a BMI of 23. She must maintain a healthy weight for pregnancy.

Signs & symptoms: Overweight, fatigue, especially after standing for a long time, lack of strength, loose stools, dizziness standing up, habitual miscarriage, severe pain and blood clots during menstruation

Tongue: Purple with raised edges and dark purple veins on the underside

Pulse: Fine, bowstring, and choppy

Pattern discrimination: Qi stagnation and blood stasis with spleen qi vacuity and phlegm dampness

Analysis of signs & symptoms: The spleen vacuity was evidenced by the fatigue, lack of strength, dizziness standing up, fine pulse, and her tendency to loose stools. In this woman's case, the habitual miscarriage was primarily due to downward falling of the central qi (complicated by blood stasis). The liver depression qi stagnation was indicated by the raised edges of the tongue and the bowstring pulse. The blood stasis was indicated by the severe dysmenorrheal, blood clots in the menstruate, and choppy pulse. Simply being overweight indicated the presence of phlegm dampness.

Treatment principles: Quicken the blood and dispel stasis, supplement and move the qi, transform phlegm and eliminate dampness

Acupuncture:

> *Tai Chong* (Liv 3) and *He Gu* (LI 4) to course the liver and rectify the qi, remembering that the qi moves the blood
> *San Yin Jiao* (Sp 6), *Xue Hai* (Sp 10), *Guan Yuan* (CV 4), and *He Gu* to quicken the blood and dispel stasis
> *Zu San Li* (St 36), *San Yin Jiao*, and *Zhong Wan* (CV 12) to fortify the spleen and supplement the qi
> *Feng Long* (St 40) and *Zhong Wan* to transform phlegm and eliminate dampness

Chinese medicinals: *Tao Hong Si Wu Tang Wan* (Persica & Carthamus Four Materials Decoction Pills), *Bu Zhong Yi Qi Wan* (Supplement the Center & Boost the Qi Pills), and *Er Chen Wan* (Two Aged [Ingredients] Pills)

Tao Hong Si Wu Tang Wan quickens the blood and dispels stasis.

Bu Zhong Yi Qi Wan fortifies the spleen, boosts the qi, and lifts the fallen. It also helps course the liver and rectify the qi.

Er Chen Wan transforms phlegm and eliminates dampness. It also helps to rectify the qi.

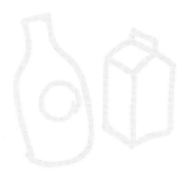

Appendix A
Chinese Medical
Food Descriptions

This appendix contains an exhaustive list of foods classified according to their thermal nature. I originally published this information on my website www.amazinghealing.com in my article "How to Treat Spleen Qi Vacuity with Medicinal Food." Since then, I have made some modifications to that original content.

Yang supplements help to warm the spleen and kidneys and move the qi, blood, and body fluids. They maintain and improve our ability to generate warmth and stimulate our system. Yang supplements include:

Basil	Fennel	Raspberry
Beef	Fenugreek seed	Rosemary
Cayenne	Garlic	Sage
Chestnut	Dried ginger	Savoy lettuce
Chive	Jasmine tea	Shrimp & prawn
Cinnamon	Lamb	Star anise
Clove	Lobster	Thyme
Crayfish	Nutmeg	Walnut
Dill seed	Pistachio	

The movement of qi is stimulated by the acrid flavor. Foods which move the qi are called qi-rectifiers in Chinese medicine. Some commonly eatern qi-rectifies include:

Basil	Coriander	Peppermint
Caraway	Dill	Radish
Cardamom	Garlic	Spearmint
Carrot	Jasmine tea	Star anise
Cayenne	Marjoram	Tangerine peel
Chive	Mustard leaf	Turmeric
Clove	Orange peel	

Cold conditions in general are improved by warming foods. In chronic cases, warm, sweet, and acrid foods are used to warm us steadily. In acute cases, warm or even hot foods are combined with stronger acrid-flavored to drive out the cold. (See the rest of this appendix for an exhaustive list of warming foods.) Warming foods include:

Anchovy	Dill	Nutmeg	Sweet potato
Basil	Fennel	Oat	Sweet rice
Bay leaf	Garlic	Onion	Trout
Black pepper	Ginger	Peach	Turnip
Coconut	Kohlrabi	Quinoa	Vinegar
Cayenne	Lamb	Rosemary	Walnut
Cherry	Leek	Scallion	Wine
Chestnut	Mussel	Shrimp	
Chicken	Mustard leaf	Spelt	
Coriander	Mutton	Squash	

Dampness results from the body's failure to move and transform fluids. Dampness is treated in Chinese medicine by two main methods. One can use acrid, aromatic, warm foods to dry or transform dampness or bland foods to seep dampness. Effective dampness-eliminating foods include:

Adzuki bean	Garlic	Onion
Alfalfa	Green tea	Parsley
Anchovy	Horseradish	Papaya
Amaranth	Jasmine tea	Pumpkin
Barley	Kidney bean	Radish
Buckwheat	Kohlrabi	Rice bran
Celery	Lemon	Rye
Corn	Mackerel	Scallion
Cranberry	Marjoram	Turnip
Daikon radish	Mushroom (button)	Umeboshi plum
Eel	Mustard leaf	

Some foods exacerbate the tendency towards dampness and should be reduced by people with damp conditions. These foods include:

Dairy products (sheep and goat products are less dampening)	Beer
	Bananas
	Sugar and sweeteners
Fatty cuts of pork, chicken, beef, duck	Saturated fats
	Greasy, fried, oily foods
Concentrated juices especially orange	Iced or cooled beverages
	Uncooked vegetables and salads
White refined wheat, bread, pasta	Tomatoes
Yeast	Oranges

Phlegm is congealed from dampness. Phlegm-transforming foods include:

Almond	Marjoram	Pear
Apple peel	Mushroom (button)	Radish
Clam	Mustard leaf	Seaweed
Daikon radish	Mustard seed	Shitake mushroom
Garlic	Olive	Shrimp
Grapefruit	Onion	
Lemon peel	Orange peel	

Appendix B
Food Energetics

GRAINS

FOOD	TEMPERATURE
Amaranth	Cool
Barley	Cool
Buckwheat	Cool
Corn	Neutral
Corn Meal	Neutral
Flax	Neutral
Glutinous Rice	Warm
Job's Tears/ Pearl Barley	Cool
Linseed	Neutral
Maize	Neutral
Millet	Cool
Non-Glutinous Rice	Neutral
Oats	Warm
Quinoa	Warm
Rice	Neutral
Rice (brown)	Neutral
Rice (sweet)	Warm
Rice (white)	Cool
Rice Bran	Neutral
Rye	Neutral
Sorghum	Warm
Spelt	Warm
Wheat	Cool
Wheat Bran	Cool

HERBS & SPICES

FOOD	TEMPERATURE	FOOD	TEMPERATURE
Aniseed	Warm	Juniper	Warm
Basil	Warm	Licorice	Neutral
Bay	Warm	Marjoram	Cool
Bell Pepper	Warm	Mint	Cool
Caraway	Warm	Mustard	Hot
Cardamon	Warm	Nettle	Cool
Carob	Warm	Nutmeg	Warm
Cayenne	Hot	Oregano	Warm
Chili	Hot	Parsley	Warm
Chive Leaf	Warm	Pepper (black)	Hot
Chive Seed	Warm	Pepper (sichuan)	Hot
Cinnamon	Hot	Pepper (white)	Hot
Cinnamon Bark	Hot	Peppermint	Cool
Cinnamon Twig	Warm	Pomelo	Cool
Clove	Warm	Purslane	Cold
Coriander	Neutral	Rosemary	Warm
Cumin	Warm	Saffron	Neutral
Dill Seed	Warm	Sage	Warm
Fennel Seed	Warm	Savoy	Warm
Fenugreek Seed	Warm	Spearmint	Warm
Garlic	Hot	Tamarind	Cool
Ginger (dry)	Hot	Thyme	Warm
Ginger (fresh)	Warm	Turmeric	Warm
Hawthorn	Warm	Umeboshi	Warm
Horseradish	Hot		

BEANS

FOOD	TEMPERATURE
Aduki Bean	Neutral
Black Bean	Warm
Black-Eyed Pea	Neutral
Broad Bean (fava)	Neutral
Chickpea	Neutral
Garbanzo/Chickpea	Cool
Green Bean	Warm
Kidney Bean	Neutral
Kidney Bean (red)	Neutral
Lentil	Neutral
Lima Bean	Cool
Mung Bean	Cool
Navy/Great Northern	Cool
Pea	Neutral
Pink Bean	Neutral
Pinto Bean	Cool
Soya Bean	Cool
Soya Bean (black)	Neutral
Soybean (black)	Neutral
Soybean (yellow)	Cool
String Bean	Neutral
Tofu	Cool

VEGETABLES & HERBS

FOOD	TEMPERATURE	FOOD	TEMPERATURE
Alfalfa Sprout	Cool	Maitake, Reishi	Cold
Amaranth (3 colored)	Cold	Mungbean Sprout	Cold
Artichoke	Cool	Mushroom (black)	Neutral
Asparagus	Cold	Mushroom (button)	Cool
Balsam Pear	Cold	Mushroom (oyster)	Warm
Bamboo Shoot	Cold	Mushroom (Portobello)	Neutral
Beets	Cool	Mushroom (white)	Cool
Bell Pepper	Warm	Mustard Green	Warm
Bok Choy	Cool	Mustard Leaf	Warm
Broccoli	Cool	Nori	Cold
Burdock Root (Gobo)	Cool	Olive	Neutral
Cabbage	Cool	Olive (Russian)	Warm
Caper	Warm	Onion	Warm
Carrot	Cool	Parsnip	Warm
Cassava/Yucca	Neutral	Plaintain	Warm
Cauliflower	Cool	Potato	Cool
Celery	Cool	Pumpkin	Warm
Chicory	Cool	Radish	Cool
Chinese Cabbage	Cold	Scallion	Warm
Chinese Chive	Warm	Seaweed	Cold
Chinese Wolfberry	Cool	Seaweed (laver)	Cold
Cucumber	Cool	Shitake Mushroom	Neutral
Daikon (mooli)	Cool	Snow Pea	Cold
Dandelion Leaf	Cold	Soybean Sprout	Cool
Eggplant	Cool	Spinach	Cool
Fungus (black)	Neutral	Spinach (water)	Cold
Fungus (hedgehog)	Neutral	Spring Onion	Warm
Fungus (white)	Neutral	Summer Squash	Warm
Gourd	Cold	Sweet Potato	Cool
Gourd (towel)	Cool	Swiss Chard	Neutral
Gourd (wax)	Cold	Taro Root	Neutral
Green Bean	Warm	Tremella	Cool
Kale	Warm	Turnip	Cold
Kelp	Cool	Water Chestnut	Warm
Kohlrabi	Neutral	Watercress	Neutral
Leek	Warm	Winter Melon	Cool
Lettuce	Cool	Winter Squash	Cool
Lotus Rhizone	Cool	Zucchini	Warm
Lotus Root	Cool		

NUTS & SEEDS

FOOD	TEMPERATURE
Almond	Neutral
Almond (sweet)	Neutral
Caraway Seed	Warm
Chestnut	Warm
Coconut	Warm
Coconut Milk	Warm
Flax	Neutral
Ginko Nut	Neutral
Hazel (filbert)	Neutral
Lotus Seed	Neutral
Peanut	Neutral
Pine Kernel	Warm
Pine Nut	Warm
Pistachio	Neutral
Pumpkin Seed	Neutral
Sesame	Neutral
Sesame (black)	Neutral
Sesame (brown)	Neutral
Sesame (white)	Neutral
Sunflower Seed	Neutral
Walnut	Warm
Winter Melon Seed	Cool

OILS, CONDIMENTS & MISCELLANEOUS

FOOD	TEMPERATURE
Agar	Cold
Amasake	Warm
Black Pepper	Warm
Brown Sugar	Warm
Chrysanthemum	Cool
Cilantro Leaf	Warm
Cinnamon	Warm
Clove	Warm
Coconut Milk	Neutral
Coriander Seed	Neutral
Honey	Neutral
Kudzu	Warm
Liquor	Cool
Malt Sugar	Neutral
Maltose	Warm
Miso	Neutral
Molasses	Hot
Olive Oil	Warm
Peanut Oil	Warm
Pepper (cayenne)	Hot
Rice Syrup	Hot
Rose	Cool
Salt	Warm
Sesame Oil	Warm
Seville Orange Flower	Warm
Soya Oil	Warm
Soya Sauce	Hot
Table Salt	Cool
Vinegar	Cold
Vinegar (rice)	Cool
White Sugar	Neutral

FISH

FOOD	TEMPERATURE
Abalone	Neutral
Anchovy	Warm
Anchovy (long-tailed)	Neutral
Butterfish	Neutral
Carp	Neutral
Carp (black)	Neutral
Carp (gran)	Warm
Carp (silver)	Neutral
Catfish	Neutral
Clam	Cold
Crab	Cold
Crayfish	Warm
Crucian Carp	Neutral
Cutterfish	Neutral
Eel	Warm
Eel (finless)	Warm
Frog	Cold
Hairtail	Warm
Herring	Neutral
Loach	Neutral
Lobster	Warm
Mackerel	Neutral
Mandarin Fish	Neutral
Mullet (snake-head)	Cold
Mussel	Warm
Octopus	Cold
Oyster	Neutral
Perch	Neutral
River Snail	Cold
Salmon	Neutral
Sardine	Neutral
Scallion	Warm
Sea Cucumber	Warm
Shark	Neutral
Shrimp (freshwater)	Warm
Shrimp/Prawn	Warm
Soft-Shelled Turtle	Neutral
Squid	Cold
Sturgeon	Neutral
Sturgeon (huso)	Neutral
Trout	Hot
Whitebait	Neutral
Whitefish	Neutral
Yellow Croaker	Neutral

FRUIT

FOOD	TEMPERATURE	FOOD	TEMPERATURE
Apple	Cool	Mango	Cool
Apricot	Neutral	Melon	Cold
Arhat (lou han)	Cool	Mulberry	Cold
Avocado	Cool	Orange	Cool
Banana	Cold	Orange (cantonese)	Cool
Blackberry	Warm	Orange (peel)	Cool
Blackcurrant	Cool	Papaya	Neutral
Blue/Bilberry	Warm	Peach	Warm
Canteloupe	Cold	Pear	Cool
Cherry	Warm	Pear (apple)	Cold
Chinese Olive	Cool	Persimmon	Cold
Coconut	Warm	Pineapple	Neutral
Cranberry	Cold	Plum	Neutral
Date	Warm	Plum (mume)	Neutral
Date (red)	Warm	Pomegranate	Neutral
Fig	Neutral	Prune (Chinese)	Warm
Grape	Warm	Quince	Warm
Grapefruit	Cold	Raspberry	Warm
Grapefruit (peel)	Warm	Red Bay Berry	Neutral
Guava	Warm	Rhubarb	Cold
Hawthorn Berry	Warm	Rosehip	Cool
Japanese Rasin Tree	Neutral	Strawberry	Cool
Kiwi	Cold	Sugar Cane	Cold
Kumquat	Warm	Tamarind	Cool
Lemon/Lime	Cool	Tangerine	Warm
Litchi	Warm	Tomato	Cool
Longan	Warm	Water Chestnut	Cold
Loquat	Neutral	Water Melon	Cold
Lychee	Warm		

BEVERAGES

FOOD	TEMPERATURE
Barley Malt Syrup	Neutral
Beer	Cool
Chamomile	Cool
Chrysanthemum	Cool
Coffee	Warm
Dandelion Root	Cold
Elderflower	Cool
Jasmine	Warm
Lemon Balm	Cool
Limeflower	Cool
Peppermint	Cool
Raspberry Leaf	Cool
Rosehip	Neutral
Soya Milk	Neutral
Star Anise	Warm
Black Tea	Slightly Warm
Green Tea	Cool
Wine	Warm
Oolong Tea	Cool

MEAT

FOOD	TEMPERATURE
Beef	Warm
Calf's (brain)	Cool
Chicken	Warm
Chicken (black-boned)	Neutral
Duck	Neutral
Frog	Cool
Goose	Neutral
Ham	Warm
Kidney (beef)	Warm
Kidney (pork)	Neutral
Kidney (sheep)	Warm
Lamb	Hot
Lamb (kidney)	Warm
Lamb (liver)	Cool
Liver (beef)	Neutral
Liver (chicken)	Warm
Liver (pork)	Warm
Liver (sheep)	Cool
Mutton	Warm
Pheasant	Warm
Pork	Cool
Quail	Neutral
Rabbit	Cool
Turkey	Warm
Vension	Warm

DAIRY

FOOD	TEMPERATURE
Butter	Warm
Cheese	Neutral
Egg (chicken)	Neutral
Egg (duck)	Neutral
Egg White (chicken)	Neutral
Egg Yoke (chicken)	Neutral
Milk (cow's not treated with antibiotics)	Neutral
Milk (cow's treated with antibiotics)	Cool
Milk (human)	Warm
Milk (sheep/goat)	Warm
Quail (eggs)	Neutral
Yogurt	Cool

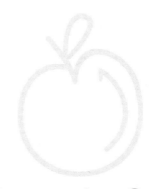

Appendix C
Medication-induced Weight Gain

Many medications are known to cause weight gain which makes weight loss very hard, if not impossible regardless of diet and lifestyle. Once the practitioner discovers that a patient's medication may be causing weight gain or precluding weight loss, do not advise the patient to stop the drug, but do advise that the patient speak with the prescribing doctor about the most safe and effective way to switch to another drug.

This appendix lists many medications and medication types which have been linked to weight gain, the vast majority of which are antidepressant selective serotonin reuptake inhibitors (SSRIs). However, selective serotonin norepinephrine reuptake inhibitors (SSNRIs) have not been linked to weight gain. Interestingly, the weight loss drug Merida is also an SSNRI. Because drug information is rapidly changing, this list of drugs which are linked to weight gain is not an exhaustive list; therefore, the reader should stay abreast of the most recent research available.

Antidepressants and SSRIs: Prozac®, Zoloft®, Paxil®, lithium, Remeron®, Zeprexa®

Anticonvulsant: Valproate®

Antipsychotic: Clozaril®

Anti-migraine: Triptans

Antihypertensive: Terazosin®

Diabetic: Some cause weight gain but some studies show that Glucophage®
combined with some of the antidepressants which cause weight
gain may actually help patients lose weight or prevent further
weight gain.

Hormone therapy: Oral birth control pills, Tamoxifen®

Insomnia medication: Ambien® has been linked to unconscious eating
during sleep.

Bibliography

Atkins, Robert, Dr. (2002). *Dr. Atkins' New Diet Revolution*. New York, NY: M. Evans and Company

Agatston, Arthur. (2003). *The South Beach Diet*. :Emmaus, PA: Rodale

Bensky, Dan & Barolet, Randall., (1990). *Chinese Herbal Medicine: Formulas and Strategies*. Seattle, WA: Eastland Press

Bensky, Dan & Clavey, Stoger, (2004). *Chinese Herbal Medicine: Materia Medica*. Seattle, WA: Eastland Press

Brand-Miller, J., Burani, J., Foster-Powell, K. (2001). *The Glucose Revolution Life Plan*. New York, NY: Marlowe & Co.

Brody, Jane E., "The Widening of America, or How Size 4 Became Size 0," *New York Times*. 20 Jan. 2004, 3A

Chang, Stephen. (1987). *The Tao of Balanced Diet*. Reno, NV: Tao Publishing

Clavey, Steven. (2003). *Fluid Physiology & Pathology in Traditional Chinese Medicine*. UK: Churchill Livingstone

Colbin, Anne Marie. (1986). *Food and Healing*. New York NY: Ballantine

Colbin, Anne Marie. (1998). *Calcium and Our Bones.* New York, NY: Plume

Deadman, Peter, & Mazin, Baker. (2001). *A Manual of Acupuncture.* East Sussex, London: Journal of Chinese Medicine Publications

Flaws, Bob. (1999). *260 Essential Chinese Medicinals.* Boulder, CO: Blue Poppy Press

Flaws, Bob. (1998). *The Tao of Healthy Eating.* Boulder, CO: Blue Poppy Press

Flaws, Bob. "New Approaches to the Chinese Medical Treatment of Obesity," *Acupuncture Today.* October 2002, Vol. 03, Issue 10

Flaws, Bob & Finney, Daniel. (1996). *A Handbook of TCM Patterns & Their Treatments.* Boulder, CO: Blue Poppy Press

Foster, Helen. (2004). *The Good Carb Diet Plan.* New York, NY: Hamlyn

Gallop, Rick. (2002). *Glycemic Index Diet.* New York, NY: Workman Publishing

Hirschman, Jane K. & Munter, Carol H. (1988). *Overcoming Overeating.* New York, NY: Ballantine

Hirschman, Jane K. & Munter, Carol H. (1995). *When Women Stop Hating Their Bodies: Freeing Yourself From Food and Weight Obsession.* New York, NY: Ballantine

Jilin, Liu & Peck, Gordon (Eds.). (2000). *Chinese Dietary Therapy.* Hong Kong: China: Churchill Livingstone

Kushi, Michio & Jack, Alex. (2003). *The Macrobiotic Path to Total Health.* New York, NY: Ballantine

Netzer, Corinne T. (1992). *The Corinne T. Netzer Encyclopedia of Food Values.* New York, NY: Random House, Inc.

Ni, Maoshing & McNease Cathy. (1996). *The Tao of Nutrition.* Santa Monica, CA: Seven Star Communications

Ni, Maoshing & McNease Cathy. (2001). *Course Materials for Certification Class in Traditional Chinese Nutrition.* Santa Monica, CA: Health & Integral Living Institute

NIH. (2000) *Executive Summary: Clinical Guidelines On The Identification, Evaluation, And Treatment of Overweight And Obesity In Adults*

NIH. (2000). *Practical Guide: Identification, Evaluation and Treatment of Overweight and Obesity in Adults*

O'Connor, John & Bensky, Dan (Eds.). (1981). *Acupuncture: A Comprehensive Text.* Seattle, WA: Eastland Press

Pipher, Mary. (1997). *Hunger Pains: The Modern Woman's Tragic Quest for Thinness.* New York, NY: Ballantine

Pitchford, Paul. (1993). *Healing with Whole Foods.* (Rev. ed.) Berkeley, CA: North Atlantic Books

Pratt, Steven & Matthews Kathy. (2004). *Super Foods.* New York, NY: Harper Collins Publishing Inc.

Putnam, J., Allshouse, J., Kantor L.S. *"U.S. Food Supply Trends: More Calories, Refined Carbohydrates and Fat," Food Review.* Winter 2002, Vol. 25 Issue 3

Sandifer, Jon. (2001). *Zen and the Art of Cooking.* Naperville, Illinois: Sourcebooks, Inc.

Sears, Barry & Lawren, Bill. (1995). *The Zone.* New York, NY: Harper Collins Publishing Inc.

Taylor, Janice. (2006). *Our Lady of Weight Loss.* New York, NY: Viking Studio

Weil, Andrew. (1997). *Eating Well for Optimum Health.* New York, NY: Alfred A. Knopf

Williams, Lindsey. (2006). *Neo Soul: Taking Soul Food to a Whole Notha' Level.* New York, NY: Avery

Wiseman, Nigel & Feng Ye. (1998). *A Practical Dictionary of Chinese Medicine.* Brookline, MA: Paradigm Publications

Wolf, Naomi. (2002). *The Beauty Myth: How Images of Beauty Are Used Against Women.* New York, NY: Perennial

Yang Shou-zhong & Li Jian-yong. (1993) *Li Dong-yan's Treatise on the Spleen & Stomach.* Boulder, CO: Blue Poppy Press

Yang, Yifan. (2002). *Chinese Herbal Medicines: Comparisons and Characteristics.* Churchhill Livingstone, London

Index

CURING DEPRESSION NATURALLY WITH
CHINESE MEDICINE
by Rosa Schnyer & Bob Flaws
ISBN 0-936185-94-5
ISBN 978-0-936185-94-1

CURING FIBROMYALGIA NATURALLY WITH
CHINESE MEDICINE
by Bob Flaws
ISBN 1-891845-09-8
ISBN 978-1-891845-09-3

CURING HAY FEVER NATURALLY WITH
CHINESE MEDICINE
by Bob Flaws
ISBN 0-936185-91-0
ISBN 978-0-936185-91-0

CURING HEADACHES NATURALLY WITH
CHINESE MEDICINE
by Bob Flaws
ISBN 0-936185-95-3
ISBN 978-0-936185-95-8

CURING IBS NATURALLY WITH CHINESE
MEDICINE
by Jane Bean Oberski
ISBN 1-891845-11-X
ISBN 978-1-891845-11-6

CURING INSOMNIA NATURALLY WITH
CHINESE MEDICINE
by Bob Flaws
ISBN 0-936185-86-4
ISBN 978-0-936185-86-6

CURING PMS NATURALLY WITH CHINESE
MEDICINE
by Bob Flaws
ISBN 0-936185-85-6
ISBN 978-0-936185-85-9

DISEASES OF THE KIDNEY & BLADDER
by Hoy Ping Yee Chan, et al.
ISBN 1-891845-37-3
ISBN 978-1-891845-35-6

THE DIVINE FARMER'S MATERIA MEDICA
A Translation of the Shen Nong Ben Cao
translation by Yang Shouz-zhong
ISBN 0-936185-96-1
ISBN 978-0-936185-96-5

DUI YAO: THE ART OF COMBINING
CHINESE HERBAL MEDICINALS
by Philippe Sionneau
ISBN 0-936185-81-3
ISBN 978-0-936185-81-1

ENDOMETRIOSIS, INFERTILITY AND
TRADITIONAL CHINESE MEDICINE:
A Laywoman's Guide
by Bob Flaws
ISBN 0-936185-14-7
ISBN 978-0-936185-14-9

THE ESSENCE OF LIU FENG-WU'S
GYNECOLOGY
by Liu Feng-wu, translated by Yang Shou-zhong
ISBN 0-936185-88-0
ISBN 978-0-936185-88-0

EXTRA TREATISES BASED ON INVESTIGATION &
INQUIRY:
A Translation of Zhu Dan-xi's Ge Zhi Yu Lun
translation by Yang Shou-zhong
ISBN 0-936185-53-8
ISBN 978-0-936185-53-8

FIRE IN THE VALLEY: TCM Diagnosis & Treatment
of Vaginal Diseases
by Bob Flaws
ISBN 0-936185-25-2
ISBN 978-0-936185-25-5

FU QING-ZHU'S GYNECOLOGY
trans. by Yang Shou-zhong and Liu Da-wei
ISBN 0-936185-35-X
ISBN 978-0-936185-35-4

FULFILLING THE ESSENCE:
A Handbook of Traditional & Contemporary
Treatments for Female Infertility
by Bob Flaws
ISBN 0-936185-48-1
ISBN 978-0-936185-48-4

GOLDEN NEEDLE WANG LE-TING: A 20th
Century Master's Approach to Acupuncture
by Yu Hui-chan and Han Fu-ru, trans. by Shuai Xue-zhong
ISBN 0-936185-78-3
ISBN 978-0-936185-78-1

A HANDBOOK OF TCM PATTERNS
& THEIR TREATMENTS
by Bob Flaws & Daniel Finney
ISBN 0-936185-70-8
ISBN 978-0-936185-70-5

A HANDBOOK OF TRADITIONAL
CHINESE DERMATOLOGY
by Liang Jian-hui, trans. by Zhang Ting-liang
& Bob Flaws
ISBN 0-936185-46-5
ISBN 978-0-936185-46-0

A HANDBOOK OF TRADITIONAL
CHINESE GYNECOLOGY
by Zhejiang College of TCM, trans. by Zhang Ting-liang
& Bob Flaws
ISBN 0-936185-06-6 (4th edit.)
ISBN 978-0-936185-06-4

A HANDBOOK OF CHINESE HEMATOLOGY
by Simon Becker
ISBN 1-891845-16-0
ISBN 978-1-891845-16-1

A HANDBOOK of TCM PEDIATRICS
by Bob Flaws
ISBN 0-936185-72-4
ISBN 978-0-936185-72-9

THE HEART & ESSENCE OF DAN-XI'S
METHODS OF TREATMENT
by Xu Dan-xi, trans. by Yang Shou-zhong
ISBN 0-926185-50-3
ISBN 978-0-936185-50-7

HERB TOXICITIES & DRUG INTERACTIONS:
A Formula Approach
by Fred Jennes with Bob Flaws
ISBN 1-891845-26-8
ISBN 978-1-891845-26-0

IMPERIAL SECRETS OF HEALTH & LONGEVITY
by Bob Flaws
ISBN 0-936185-51-1
ISBN 978-0-936185-51-4

INSIGHTS OF A SENIOR ACUPUNCTURIST
by Miriam Lee
ISBN 0-936185-33-3
ISBN 978-0-936185-33-0

INTEGRATED PHARMACOLOGY: Combining Modern
Pharmacology with Chinese Medicine
by Dr. Greg Sperber with Bob Flaws
ISBN 1-891845-41-1
ISBN 978-0-936185-41-3

INTRODUCTION TO THE USE OF
PROCESSED CHINESE MEDICINALS
by Philippe Sionneau
ISBN 0-936185-62-7
ISBN 978-0-936185-62-0

KEEPING YOUR CHILD HEALTHY WITH
CHINESE MEDICINE
by Bob Flaws
ISBN 0-936185-71-6
ISBN 978-0-936185-71-2

THE LAKESIDE MASTER'S STUDY OF THE PULSE
by Li Shi-zhen, trans. by Bob Flaws
ISBN 1-891845-01-2
ISBN 978-1-891845-01-7

MANAGING MENOPAUSE NATURALLY WITH
CHINESE MEDICINE
by Honora Lee Wolfe
ISBN 0-936185-98-8
ISBN 978-0-936185-98-9

MASTER HUA'S CLASSIC OF THE
CENTRAL VISCERA
by Hua Tuo, trans. by Yang Shou-zhong
ISBN 0-936185-43-0
ISBN 978-0-936185-43-9

THE MEDICAL I CHING: Oracle of the
Healer Within
by Miki Shima
ISBN 0-936185-38-4
ISBN 978-0-936185-38-5

MENOPAIUSE & CHINESE MEDICINE
by Bob Flaws
ISBN 1-891845-40-3
ISBN 978-1-891845-40-6

TEST PREP WORKBOOK FOR THE NCCAOM BIO-
MEDICINE MODULE: Exam Preparation & Study
Guide
by Zhong Bai-song
ISBN 1-891845-34-9
ISBN 978-1-891845-34-5

POINTS FOR PROFIT: The Essential Guide to
Practice Success for Acupuncturists 3rd Edition
by Honora Wolfe, Eric Strand & Marilyn Allen
ISBN 1-891845-25-X
ISBN 978-1-891845-25-3

PRINCE WEN HUI's COOK: Chinese Dietary Therapy
By Bob Flaws & Honora Wolfe
ISBN 0-912111-05-4
ISBN 978-0-912111-05-6

THE PULSE CLASSIC:
A Translation of the Mai Jing
by Wang Shu-he, trans. by Yang Shou-zhong
ISBN 0-936185-75-9
ISBN 978-0-936185-75-0

THE SECRET OF CHINESE PULSE DIAGNOSIS
by Bob Flaws
ISBN 0-936185-67-8
ISBN 978-0-936185-67-5

SECRET SHAOLIN FORMULAS for the Treatment of
External Injury
by De Chan, trans. by Zhang Ting-liang & Bob Flaws
ISBN 0-936185-08-2
ISBN 978-0-936185-08-8

STATEMENTS OF FACT IN TRADITIONAL
CHINESE MEDICINE   Revised & Expanded
by Bob Flaws
ISBN 0-936185-52-X
ISBN 978-0-936185-52-1

STICKING TO THE POINT 1:
A Rational Methodology for the Step by Step
Formulation & Administration of an Acupuncture
Treatment
by Bob Flaws
ISBN 0-936185-17-1
ISBN 978-0-936185-17-0

STICKING TO THE POINT 2:
A Study of Acupuncture & Moxibustion Formulas
and Strategies
by Bob Flaws
ISBN 0-936185-97-X
ISBN 978-0-936185-97-2

A STUDY OF DAOIST ACUPUNCTURE &
MOXIBUSTION
by Liu Zheng-cai
ISBN 1-891845-08-X
ISBN 978-1-891845-08-6

THE SUCCESSFUL CHINESE HERBALIST
by Bob Flaws and Honora Lee Wolfe
ISBN 1-891845-29-2
ISBN 978-1-891845-29-1

THE SYSTEMATIC CLASSIC OF ACUPUNCTURE
& MOXIBUSTION
A translation of the Jia Yi Jing
by Huang-fu Mi, trans. by Yang Shou-zhong &
Charles Chace
ISBN 0-936185-29-5
ISBN 978-0-936185-29-3

THE TAO OF HEALTHY EATING ACCORDING TO
CHINESE MEDICINE
by Bob Flaws
ISBN 0-936185-92-9
ISBN 978-0-936185-92-7

TEACH YOURSELF TO READ MODERN
MEDICAL CHINESE
by Bob Flaws
ISBN 0-936185-99-6
ISBN 978-0-936185-99-6

TEST PREP WORKBOOK FOR BASIC TCM THEORY
by Zhong Bai-song
ISBN 1-891845-43-8
ISBN 978-1-891845-43-7

TREATING PEDIATRIC BED-WETTING WITH
ACUPUNCTURE & CHINESE MEDICINE
by Robert Helmer
ISBN 1-891845-33-0
ISBN 978-1-891845-33-8

TREATISE on the SPLEEN & STOMACH: A
Translation and annotation of Li Dong-yuan's
Pi Wei Lun
by Bob Flaws
ISBN 0-936185-41-4
ISBN 978-0-936185-41-5

THE TREATMENT OF CARDIOVASCULAR
DISEASES WITH CHINESE MEDICINE
by Simon Becker, Bob Flaws &
Robert Casañas, MD
ISBN 1-891845-27-6
ISBN 978-1-891845-27-7

THE TREATMENT OF DIABETES MELLITUS WITH
CHINESE MEDICINE
by Bob Flaws, Lynn Kuchinski &
Robert Casañas, M.D.
ISBN 1-891845-21-7
ISBN 978-1-891845-21-5

THE TREATMENT OF DISEASE IN TCM, Vol. 1:
Diseases of the Head & Face, Including Mental &
Emotional Disorders
by Philippe Sionneau & Lü Gang
ISBN 0-936185-69-4
ISBN 978-0-936185-69-9

THE TREATMENT OF DISEASE IN TCM, Vol. II:
Diseases of the Eyes, Ears, Nose, & Throat
by Sionneau & Lü
ISBN 0-936185-73-2
ISBN 978-0-936185-73-6

THE TREATMENT OF DISEASE IN TCM, Vol. III:
Diseases of the Mouth, Lips, Tongue, Teeth & Gums
by Sionneau & Lü
ISBN 0-936185-79-1
ISBN 978-0-936185-79-8

THE TREATMENT OF DISEASE IN TCM, Vol IV:
Diseases of the Neck, Shoulders, Back, & Limbs
by Philippe Sionneau & Lü Gang
ISBN 0-936185-89-9
ISBN 978-0-936185-89-7

THE TREATMENT OF DISEASE IN TCM, Vol V:
Diseases of the Chest & Abdomen
by Philippe Sionneau & Lü Gang
ISBN 1-891845-02-0
ISBN 978-1-891845-02-4

THE TREATMENT OF DISEASE IN TCM, Vol VI:
Diseases of the Urogential System & Proctology
by Philippe Sionneau & Lü Gang
ISBN 1-891845-05-5
ISBN 978-1-891845-05-5

THE TREATMENT OF DISEASE IN TCM, Vol VII:
General Symptoms
by Philippe Sionneau & Lü Gang
ISBN 1-891845-14-4
ISBN 978-1-891845-14-7

THE TREATMENT OF EXTERNAL DISEASES
WITH ACUPUNCTURE & MOXIBUSTION
by Yan Cui-lan and Zhu Yun-long, trans. by Yang Shou-zhong
ISBN 0-936185-80-5
ISBN 978-0-936185-80-4

THE TREATMENT OF MODERN WESTERN
MEDICAL DISEASES WITH CHINESE MEDICINE
by Bob Flaws & Philippe Sionneau
ISBN 1-891845-20-9
ISBN 978-1-891845-20-8

UNDERSTANDING THE DIFFICULT PATIENT: A
Guide for Practitioners of Oriental Medicine
by Nancy Bilello, RN, L.ac.
ISBN 1-891845-32-2
ISBN 978-1-891845-32-1

YI LIN GAI CUO (Correcting the Errors in the Forest
of Medicine)
by Wang Qing-ren
ISBN 1-891845-39-X
ISBN 978-1-891845-39-0

70 ESSENTIAL CHINESE HERBAL FORMULAS
by Bob Flaws
ISBN 0-936185-59-7
ISBN 978-0-936185-59-0

160 ESSENTIAL CHINESE READY-MADE
MEDICINES
by Bob Flaws
ISBN 1-891945-12-8
ISBN 978-1-891945-12-3

630 QUESTIONS & ANSWERS ABOUT CHINESE
HERBAL MEDICINE:
A Workbook & Study Guide
by Bob Flaws
ISBN 1-891845-04-7
ISBN 978-1-891845-04-8

260 ESSENTIAL CHINESE MEDICINALS
by Bob Flaws
ISBN 1-891845-03-9
ISBN 978-1-891845-03-1

750 QUESTIONS & ANSWERS ABOUT
ACUPUNCTURE
Exam Preparation & Study Guide
by Fred Jennes
ISBN 1-891845-22-5
ISBN 978-1-891845-22-2